Controversies in Facial Plastic Surgery

Editors

FRED G. FEDOK
ROBERT M. KELLMAN

FACIAL PLASTIC SURGERY CLINICS OF NORTH AMERICA

www.facialplastic.theclinics.com

Consulting Editor
J. REGAN THOMAS

May 2018 • Volume 26 • Number 2

ELSEVIER

1600 John F. Kennedy Boulevard • Suite 1800 • Philadelphia, Pennsylvania, 19103-2899

http://www.theclinics.com

FACIAL PLASTIC SURGERY CLINICS OF NORTH AMERICA Volume 26, Number 2
May 2018 ISSN 1064-7406, ISBN-13: 978-0-323-58352-7

Editor: Jessica McCool
Developmental Editor: Sara Watkins

Facial Plastic Surgery Clinics of North America (ISSN 1064-7406) is published quarterly by Elsevier Inc., 360 Park Avenue South, New York, NY 10010-1710. Months of issue are February, May, August, and November. Business and Editorial Offices: 1600 John F. Kennedy Blvd., Suite 1800, Philadelphia, PA 19103-2899. Periodicals postage paid at New York, NY, and additional mailing offices. Subscription prices are $398.00 per year (US individuals), $628.00 per year (US institutions), $454.00 per year (Canadian individuals), $782.00 per year (Canadian institutions), $535.00 per year (foreign individuals), $782.00 per year (foreign institutions), $100.00 per year (US students), and $255.00 per year (foreign students). Foreign air speed delivery is included in all *Clinics* subscription prices. All prices are subject to change without notice. POSTMASTER: Send address changes to *Facial Plastic Surgery Clinics*, Elsevier Health Sciences Division, Subscription Customer Service, 3251 Riverport Lane, Maryland Heights, MO 63043. **Customer service: 1-800-654-2452 (US and Canada); 1-314-447-8871 (outside US and Canada); Fax: 314-447-8029; E-mail: journalscustomerservice-usa@elsevier.com (for print support); journalsonline support-usa@elsevier.com (for online support).**

Reprints. For copies of 100 or more of articles in this publication, please contact the Commercial Reprints Department, Elsevier Inc., 360 Park Avenue South, New York, NY 10010-1710. Tel.: 212-633-3874; Fax: 212-633-3820; E-mail: reprints@elsevier.com.

Facial Plastic Surgery Clinics of North America is covered in *MEDLINE/PubMed* (*Index Medicus*).

Contributors

CONSULTING EDITOR

J. REGAN THOMAS, MD
Professor, Facial Plastic and Reconstructive
Surgery, Department of Otolaryngology-Head
and Neck Surgery, Northwestern University
Feinberg School of Medicine, Chicago,
Illinois, USA

EDITORS

FRED G. FEDOK, MD, FACS
Fedok Plastic Surgery, Foley, Alabama, USA;
Adjunct Professor, Department of Surgery,
University of South Alabama, Mobile, Alabama,
USA

ROBERT M. KELLMAN, MD
Professor and Chair, Department of
Otolaryngology & Communication Sciences,
SUNY Upstate Medical University, Syracuse,
New York, USA

AUTHORS

ANURAG AGARWAL, MD, FACS
Private Practice, Naples, Florida

KOFI BOAHENE, MD, FACS
Associate Professor, Facial Plastic and
Reconstructive Surgery, Department of
Otolaryngology–Head and Neck Surgery,
Johns Hopkins Medical Institute, Baltimore,
Maryland, USA

ANTHONY E. BRISSETT, MD, FACS
Chief, Division of Facial Plastic and
Reconstructive Surgery, Acting
Associate Professor, Institute of
Academic Medicine, Houston Methodist
ENT & Facial Plastic Surgery Associates,
Houston Methodist Hospital, Huston,
Texas, USA

LISA BUNIN, MD
Oculoplastic Surgeon, Private Practice,
Allentown, Pennsylvania, USA

ANDREW CAMPBELL, MD
Quintessa Aesthetic Centers, Sheboygan,
Wisconsin, USA

PAUL J. CARNIOL, MD
Clinical Professor and Director, Facial
Plastic Surgery, Department of
Otolaryngology–Head and Neck Surgery,
Rutgers New Jersey Medical School,
Summit, New Jersey, USA

LOUIS M. DeJOSEPH, MD
Department of Otolaryngology–Head
and Neck Surgery, Clinical Instructor,
Emory University, Premier Image
Cosmetic & Laser Surgery, Atlanta,
Georgia, USA

REBECCA FITZGERALD, MD
Dermatologist, Private Practice, Los
Angeles, California, USA

OREN FRIEDMAN, MD
Associate Professor, Director, Facial
Plastic Surgery, Department of
Otorhinolaryngology–Head and Neck
Surgery, University of Pennsylvania,
Philadelphia, Pennsylvania,
USA

ANDRES GANTOUS, MD, FRCS(C), FACS
Department of Otolaryngology–Head and Neck Surgery, Division of Facial Plastic and Reconstructive Surgery, Associate Professor, University of Toronto, Toronto, Ontario, Canada

RICHARD D. GENTILE, MD, MBA
Gentile Facial Plastic and Aesthetic Laser Center, Youngstown, Ohio, USA

TIMOTHY M. GRECO, MD, FACS
Adjunct Assistant Professor, Perelman School of Medicine, University of Pennsylvania, Philadelphia, Pennsylvania, USA

LISA D. GRUNEBAUM, MD
Associate Professor, Otolaryngology–Head and Neck Surgery, University of Miami Miller School of Medicine, Miami, Florida, USA

TESSA A. HADLOCK, MD
Director, Division of Facial Plastic and Reconstructive Surgery, Director, Facial Nerve Center, Professor, Otolaryngology–Head and Neck Surgery, Massachusetts Eye and Ear Infirmary, Harvard Medical School, Boston, Massachusetts, USA

GRANT S. HAMILTON III, MD
Assistant Professor, Department of Otorhinolaryngology, Mayo Clinic, Rochester, Minnesota, USA

MARK HAMILTON, MD
Hamilton Facial Plastic Surgery, Greenwood, Indiana, USA

RYAN N. HEFFELFINGER, MD
Associate Professor, Director, Division of Facial Plastic and Reconstructive Surgery, Thomas Jefferson University Hospitals, Philadelphia, Pennsylvania, USA

J. DAVID HOLCOMB, MD
Holcomb-Kreithen Plastic Surgery and MedSpa, Sarasota, Florida, USA

NATHAN JOHNSON, MD
Private Practice, Facial Plastic and Reconstructive Surgery, Ear, Nose and Throat SpecialtyCare of Minnesota, Minneapolis, Minnesota, USA

LAMONT R. JONES, MD, MBA
Vice Chair, Department of Otolaryngology–Head and Neck Surgery, Facial Plastic and Reconstructive Surgery, Co-Director, Cleft and Craniofacial Clinic, Henry Ford Health System, Detroit, Michigan, USA

BRIAN M. KINNEY, MD, FACS, MSME
Clinical Associate Professor of Plastic Surgery, Plastic and Reconstructive Surgery, University of Southern California (USC), Beverly Hills, California, USA

THEDA C. KONTIS, MD
Associate Professor, Department of Otolaryngology–Head and Neck Surgery, Division of Facial Plastic and Reconstructive Surgery, Johns Hopkins Medical Institute, Facial Plastic Surgicenter, LLC, Baltimore, Maryland, USA

JESSYKA G. LIGHTHALL, MD
Director, Facial Plastic and Reconstructive Surgery, Assistant Professor, Department of Surgery, Division of Otolaryngology–Head and Neck Surgery, Penn State Health Milton S. Hershey Medical Center, Hershey, Pennsylvania, USA

KRIS S. MOE, MD, FACS
Professor and Chief, Division of Facial Plastic and Reconstructive Surgery, Departments of Otolaryngology and Neurological Surgery, University of Washington School of Medicine, Seattle, Washington, USA

ANDREW H. MURR, MD, FACS
Professor and Chairman, Department of Otolaryngology–Head and Surgery, University of California, San Francisco, School of Medicine, San Francisco, California, USA

JOSE CARLOS NEVES, MD
Director, My Face, Clinica da Face, Lisboa, Portugal; My Face, Clinica da Face, Coimbra, Portugal

STEPHEN W. PERKINS, MD
Private Practice, President and Founder, Meridian Plastic Surgery Center, Meridian Plastic Surgeons, Indianapolis, Indiana, USA

HARRISON C. PUTMAN III, MD
Assistant Clinical Professor, Department of
Otolaryngology, SIU School of Medicine,
Springfield, Illinois; Private Practice, Peoria,
Illinois, USA

**NEIL S. SADICK, MD, FAAD, FAACS, FACP,
FACPh**
Clinical Professor of Dermatology, Weill Cornell
Medical College, New York, New York, USA

ABEL-JAN TASMAN, MD
Rhinology, Facial Plastic Surgery, ENT
Department, Cantonal Hospital St. Gallen,
Hals-Nasen-Ohrenklinik, St Gallen,
Switzerland

TRAVIS T. TOLLEFSON, MD, MPH
Director, Facial Plastic and Reconstructive
Surgery, Professor, Department of
Otolaryngology–Head and Neck Surgery,
University of California, Davis, UC Davis
Medical Center, Sacramento, California, USA

WILLIAM H. TRUSWELL IV, MD
Private Practice, Easthampton,
Massachusetts, USA; Private Practice,
Charleston, South Carolina, USA; Clinical
Instructor, Department of Surgery, Facial
Plastic Surgery, Division of Otolaryngology,
University of Connecticut School of
Medicine, Farmington, Connecticut, USA

SARA TULLIS WESTER, MD, FACS
Associate Professor of Clinical
Ophthalmology, Oculofacial Plastic,
Reconstructive Surgery, Orbit and Oncology,
Bascom Palmer Eye Institute, University of
Miami Miller School of Medicine, Miami,
Florida, USA

BRIAN J.F. WONG, MD, PhD
Professor and Vice Chairman, Director,
Departments of Otolaryngology–Head and
Neck Surgery and Biomedical Engineering,
Division of Facial Plastic Surgery, University
of California, Irvine, Irvine, California, USA

Contents

neuromuscular training, nonsurgical management, and the future of this field. All the authors answered these questions in a "How I do it" manner to provide the reader with a true understanding of their thoughts and techniques. This article provides a practical resource to all physicians and practitioners treating patients with facial paralysis on some of the most common questions and issues.

 Video content accompanies this article at http://www.facialplastic.theclinics.com.

This article incorporates the opinions and preferred surgical options in managing patients of 3 prominent facial plastic surgeons who have large otoplasty practices. Six different questions covering the management of prominent ears are answered by the 3 practitioners. Nonsurgical options for the treatment of prominent ears are discussed. The role of cartilage-cutting and cartilage-sparing techniques, as well as individual preferred otoplasty techniques, is thoroughly covered. Postoperative management of these patients is presented by the individual surgeons.

This article examines 6 questions about lip augmentation answered by 3 experts in their field of facial plastic surgery. The topics covered include high-yield areas such as injection, surgical enhancement, rhytid resurfacing, implants, complications, and technique changes over the years. All the authors answered these questions in a "How I do it" manner to provide the reader with a true understanding of their thoughts and techniques. This article provides a practical resource to all physicians and practitioners performing lip augmentation on some of the most common questions and issues.

With the adoption of open structure techniques, rhinoplasty has become more reliant on the use of structural grafts to resist change that occurs over time owing to both gravity and the aging process. As surgical procedures have become more technically complex, the type of grafts used for both primary and secondary rhinoplasty have undergone significant evolution. This article provides a case approach focused on the use of structural grafting in rhinoplasty.

Injectable products are now being designed to treat specific areas of the face, including the lower lid and cheek region, the midface, and circumoral rhytids. Expert injectors from 3 core disciplines (facial plastic surgery, oculoplastic surgery, and dermatology) were asked to discuss their approaches to the midface, lower lid, and cheek region and their opinions about using cannulas versus needles. The authors describe their techniques for avoiding and managing filler complications. They give insight into how their techniques have changed over the past few years and their use of new products that have been developed.

Orbital Fractures   237

Kris S. Moe, Andrew H. Murr, and Sara Tullis Wester

Anatomic, rather than volumetric, reconstruction leads to improved outcomes in orbital reconstruction. Endoscopic visualization improves lighting and magnification of the surgical site and allows the entire operative team to understand and participate in the procedure. Mirror-image overlay display with navigation-guided surgery allows in situ fine adjustment of the implant contours to match the contralateral uninjured orbit. Precise exophthalmometry is important before, during, and after surgery to provide optimal surgical results.

Evaluating New Technology   253

Paul J. Carniol, Ryan N. Heffelfinger, and Lisa D. Grunebaum

There are multiple complex issues to consider when evaluating any new technology. First evaluate the efficacy of the device. Then considering your patient population, decide whether this technology brings an added benefit to your patients. If it meets these 2 criteria, then proceed to the financial analysis of acquiring this technology. The complete financial analysis has several important components that include but are not limited to cost, value, alternatives, return on investment, and associated marketing expense.

FACIAL PLASTIC SURGERY CLINICS OF NORTH AMERICA

THE CLINICS ARE AVAILABLE ONLINE!
Access your subscription at:
www.theclinics.com

Preface
Controversies in Facial Plastic Surgery

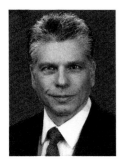 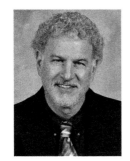

Fred G. Fedok, MD, FACS   Robert M. Kellman, MD

Editors

Over the last 50+ years, the field of facial plastic surgery has evolved into a prominent subspecialty in surgery. This discipline encompasses the care of the entire region of the face, scalp, and neck. With the professional evolution of the field, there has also been an evolution and growth of the knowledge base of facial plastic surgery. The field lends expertise, understanding, and direction in all facets of the regional reconstructive, corrective, and cosmetic concerns.

This consolidation and maturation of the field are due to the development of several generations of experts in facial plastic surgery. This has been possible through extensive avenues of education, training, and experience. There are experts in free tissue transfer, in vascular disorders, in the management of scars, rhinoplasty, related technology, and aging face surgery, as well as in every other concern that is of interest in the region.

Salient questions were selected by the authors and the editors that allowed the authors to expound on their particular approaches and viewpoints. In some cases, various experts agreed, and in others, differed. The variation of views allows the reader to compare answers and come to their own conclusions.

These experts practice in a variety of settings: they practice as academic faculty and chairs, they practice as solo practitioners, and they practice as members of large and well-recognized multispecialty groups. As this interconnected body of facial plastic surgeons, they teach, disseminate knowledge, and benefit the patients around them. Facial Plastic Surgery now has an expanding worldwide footprint.

This issue of *Facial Plastic Surgery Clinics of North America* is the third in a series of panel discussions. The purpose of this format, as produced and edited by Elsevier, is to be reflective of some of the current issues facing facial plastic surgeons practicing in a variety of settings. Timely questions have been developed through the interview of experts in the various realms presented. It is intended to allow the reading audience to enjoy the varying opinions and practices of the authors. All are well-known experts in the respective realms of facial plastic surgery they are commenting on. We believe the readers will find the comments and responses helpful in their own practices.

As the editors of this issue, we would like to thank the authors who accepted the challenge of selecting the panel of authors for the respective articles: You have done well. This group of experts has created the awesome value of this issue.

Finally, to the readers, we trust you will find this to be an enjoyable read thanks to the expert editing of the Elsevier personnel. Enclosed you will find the answers to many day-to-day and

Facial Plast Surg Clin N Am 26 (2018) xi–xii
https://doi.org/10.1016/j.fsc.2017.12.012
1064-7406/18/© 2017 Published by Elsevier Inc.

"big" questions you may encounter in your practices.

Be well and best regards,

Fred G. Fedok, MD, FACS
Fedok Plastic Surgery
113 East Fern Avenue
Foley, AL 36535, USA

Department of Surgery
University of South Alabama
Mobile, AL 36617, USA

Robert M. Kellman, MD
Department of Otolaryngology &
Communication Sciences
SUNY–Upstate Medical University
750 East Adams Street
Syracuse, NY 13210, USA

E-mail addresses:
drfredfedok@me.com (F.G. Fedok)
kellmanr@upstate.edu (R.M. Kellman)

Facial Plastic Surgery Controversies: Keloids

Kofi Boahene, MD[a], Anthony E. Brissett, MD[b], Lamont R. Jones, MD, MBA[c,*]

KEYWORDS

• Keloid • Fibroproliferative tumor • Keloid treatment • Keloid risk factors • Keloid prophylaxis

KEY POINTS

- The 3 main barriers to improved keloid treatment outcomes are incomplete understanding of keloid pathogenesis and lack of biomarkers and animal models.
- Keloid risk factors vary by site in the head and neck, and its incidence after head and neck surgery may be lower than reported for other areas.
- The prophylactic treatment of known keloid formers should include a perioperative plan to minimize inflammation, cellular proliferation, and wound tension.
- Keloids are a chronic condition that requires proper disease education and long-term follow-up.
- There are no clear indications for radiation therapy for keloid treatment but it is generally reserved for recurrence, and its usage should be balanced with radiation safety and effectiveness.

Panel discussion

1. What are the barriers to better outcomes for keloid treatment?

2. What are risk factors for keloids in otolaryngology patients?

3. What is your prophylactic protocol for treating known keloid formers?

4. How long do you treat or follow patients after surgical removal?

5. When do you consider radiation therapy for the management of keloids?

6. What is your prophylactic protocol when operating on known keloid formers?

Question 1: What are the barriers to better outcomes for keloid treatment?

JONES

For the more than 11 million people in the world affected with keloids,[1] the goals for better treatment outcomes are evident. I believe patients want return of form and function, respite from physical symptoms and emotional distress,[2] and more reliable results with lower recurrence rates without concomitant treatment mortality and nominal morbidity. I perceive 3 main barriers to improved outcomes for keloid treatment. First, incomplete understanding of keloid pathogenesis; second, lack of biomarkers; and third, the absence of an acceptable animal model.

Disclosure Statement: The authors have nothing to disclose.
[a] Facial Plastic and Reconstructive Surgery, Department of Otolaryngology–Head and Neck Surgery, Johns Hopkins Medical Institute, 601 North Caroline Street, Baltimore, MD 21287, USA; [b] Division of Facial Plastic and Reconstructive Surgery, Institute of Academic Medicine, Houston Methodist ENT and Facial Plastic Surgery Associates, Houston Methodist Hospital, 6550 Fannin Street, Suite 1703, Huston, TX 77030, USA; [c] Department of Otolaryngology–Head and Neck Surgery, Henry Ford Health Hospital, 2799 West Grand Boulevard, Detroit, MI 48202, USA
* Corresponding author.
E-mail address: Ljones5@hfhs.org

Facial Plast Surg Clin N Am 26 (2018) 105–112
https://doi.org/10.1016/j.fsc.2017.12.001

Keloids are fibroproliferative tumors that occur after injury to the skin. Their pathogenesis is characterized by overgrowth, which is the result of hyperplasia and increased amounts of extracellular matrix, secondary to increased proliferation and activity of several cell types in the keloid microenvironment.[3] Fibroblasts have been identified as a key player in the pathogenesis of keloids, but the drivers are unkown.[4,5] Moreover, other cell types, such as keratinocytes, play a role through paracrine regulation of fibroblast function.[6] Genetic studies have identified genes that explain only part of the biological or functional changes associated with keloids.[7] Epigenetics, the study of changes in gene expression that occur without changing the DNA sequence, may provide a new direction for the study of keloid pathogenesis.[7] It has been postulated that keloid disease is influenced by aberrant signaling pathways.[8] Research has focused on cytokines, such as transforming growth factor-β and epidermal growth factor, given their implications in other fibrotic disease.[3,9] No clear signaling pathway, however, has been identified. Despite the increased focus on keloid pathogenesis, current approaches of research have yielded some tangible results, albeit with large gaps in understanding of keloid pathogenesis.[4] Overall, a better understanding of the heterogeneity of the mechanisms of keloid formation will allow for development of potential novel therapies for improved treatment outcomes.

Biomarkers identify the presence of disease and can be used for diagnosis and clinical and translational research outcomes. The lack of keloid biomarkers prevents standardized and reproducible data that can be objectively evaluated and compared. For example, keloids and hypertrophic scars are not always easy to differentiate, despite research describing in detail the clinical and morphologic differences.[5] Biomarkers play a critical role in improving drug development[6] and subsequent outcomes for therapy. There are no Food and Drug Administration–approved therapies to treat keloids. Current treatment options are fraught with unacceptable recurrence rates. Nevertheless, some patients benefit from multimodality therapies. Keloid biomarkers would allow for better prediction of outcomes and weighing of risks and benefits of treatment options. Moreover, they would serve as targets and allow for precision therapies that take into account the heterogeneity in keloid formation.

Animal models are also needed to help improve keloid outcomes. Keloids occur only in humans.[7] Current in vitro methods to study keloids do not account for their complexity.[9] Animal models aid in elucidating underlying mechanisms of disease and allow for therapeutic interventions to be studied in a controlled environment.[10] They often represent the last preclinical step in the therapeutic pipeline of translational research. Despite the existence of several animal models to study wound healing, fibrosis, and scarring, none is specific to keloids. Moreover, current in vitro and in vivo models cannot explain why wound healing results in normal, hypertrophic, or keloid scar formation. Better outcomes in keloid treatment will hasten with the advent of an acceptable animal model.

BOAHNENE

Over several decades, keloid treatment failure has remained high and present outcomes are overall unsatisfactory. The quest for better outcomes underlies the wide-ranging variation in treatment regimens and recommendations. Inadequate research funding is always suggested as an impediment to medical discovery and treatment progress and this may be true for keloids. There are, however, additional barriers to understanding keloids and achieving better treatment outcomes. First, keloids are classified as scars that cause mainly cosmetic deformities. As such they do not attract the focused clinical attention necessary to generate significant breakthrough. There are no "centers of keloid treatment" that I am aware of. Perhaps the classification of keloids as mere scars that grow beyond their original boundary should be revisited. Clinically, keloids vary in their behavior but are generally locally aggressive processes capable of replacing normal tissue not so dissimilar to certain neoplastic processes. A change in approach from scar management to treatment of aggressive soft tissue tumor may be necessary to bend the curve in treatment outcomes. Second, there is a major gap in translating the understandings gained from elucidating the pathogenesis of keloid formation from the molecular level to clinical practice. One major reason for this is the lack of an animal keloid model that will allow experimental targeting of potential steps in the disease pathways. Tissue engineering techniques that seek to replicate disease processes ex vivo are shortening the testing of newly developed pharmaceutical products. As desirable replacement of animal experiments, tissue-engineered skin equivalents have recently been applied in microbial and viral infection models. A similar approach to the study of keloids and effectiveness of new therapies holds promise.

BRISSETT

The barriers to improved outcomes for patients suffering from keloids are multifactorial and often centered around the poorly understood pathogenesis of this proliferative process. Additionally, the lack of reliable treatment protocols limits standardized treatments and minimizes reliable and predictable outcomes. Finally, patients are often unaware of the signs and symptoms that herald the onset of recurrence and reactivation. The lack of awareness of signs and symptoms of reactivation often results in patients presenting for treatment late in the face of recurrence, thus limiting the effectiveness of treatment outcomes.

Question 2: What are risk factors for keloids in otolaryngology patients?

JONES

Keloids account for more than 425,000 clinic visits yearly in the United States.[11] The main risk factor for development of keloids is injury to the skin dermal layer, including surgery, in at-risk individuals. The incidence is up to 15% to 20% in patients with darker skin.[7] In addition, those who develop keloids tend to have a family history of keloids and are younger.[12] Although few studies have assessed risk factors for keloids in otolaryngology patients, the incidence after head and neck surgery may be lower than that reported for other sites.[7] Patients frequently present to an otolaryngologist for treatment of keloids after ear piercing. There is an increased incidence of ear keloids with increased popularity of piercings. Also, there is an increase in ear keloids when ear piercings occur after age 11 years and more so in those with a family history.[13] Other risk factors for keloids in otolaryngology patients include increased wound tension, delayed wound healing, and regional susceptibility, such as periauricular, cheek, scalp, and beard areas.[14,15] Pseudofolliculitis barbae and ace keloidalis nuchae are also causes of keloid formation in the head and neck area. Pseudofolliculitis barbae is a condition caused by foreign body reaction to ingrown hairs in the beard area. This usually occurs after shaving in individuals with coarse and curly hair, most commonly African American men. It can also occur with cheek and chin hair were hair plucking is a common cause.[16] An inflammatory reaction to the hair leads to microabscess in the epidermis and eventual abscess formation and giant cell reaction in the dermis.[17] Keloidalis nuchae is a condition characterized by papule and plaque-like keloid lesions in the nape of the neck and posterior scalp. Similar to pseudofolliculitis barbae, it is caused by chronic inflammation as a result of folliculitis. Acne is also a cause of keloid formation, mainly in the cheek area. Similar to the initiation of acne, there is an increased incidence of keloid formation after ear piercing, pseudofolliculitis barbae, and keloidalis nuchae after the onset of puberty.

BOAHENE

In my practice, the common sites for keloid formation in the head and neck region are ear lobe, posterior auricular region, occipital scalp, and upper neck. Earlobe keloids commonly result from late ear piercing. I have encountered periauricular keloids that have resulted from surgical incisions for mastoidectomy, paroticedtomy, and ear cartilage harvest. Keloids in hair-bearing and bearded areas are thought to result from ingrown hair. Clinicians should consider prophylactic measures to reduce the risk for keloid formation when operating in the high-risk areas (discussed previously) in high-risk patients.

BRISSETT

The head and neck area represents the region most commonly affected by hypertrophic scars and keloids. The primary risk factor related to the development of keloids is a history of epidermal and dermal injury. People of color, Africans, Hispanics, and Asian are at increased risk for developing keloids. The earlobe is the most commonly affected area in the head and neck region and is believed to be the result of ear piercing. Although piercing may be the inciting traumatic event in many of these scenarios the earlobe keloid often develops after an infection or inflammatory response of the surrounding soft tissue envelope and then subsequent removal of the earring itself. In addition to the trauma caused by the act of piercing, removal of the earring results in trapped epidermal and dermal elements inciting further inflammation and increased fibroblast proliferation.

Question 3: What is your prophylactic protocol for treating known keloid formers?

BRISSETT

The prophylactic treatment of known keloid formers often begins during the preoperative phase. When treating a patient with an active keloid, the primary focus for treating the keloid patient preoperatively is to minimize the inflammatory and proliferative aspects of the keloid; this is most often accomplished with the use combination treatments, such as antihistamines; intralesional injections, such as triamcinolone and 5- fluorouracil (5-FU); and topical treatments, such as silicone sheeting and other occlusive style dressings. The implementation of a comprehensive preoperative management protocol for patients with active keloids allows the surgeon to determine the responsiveness of keloids to treatment and increases the likelihood of selecting the best postsurgical treatment plan.[1] In many cases, the preoperative treatment of keloids can relieve the symptoms of keloids and thus obviate surgical intervention.

Once a decision has been made to move forward with a surgical procedure on a known or suspected keloid former, judicious and appropriate placement of incisions and meticulous attention to surgical technique are paramount. During the surgical planning phase, the placement of incisions within relaxed skin tension lines or facial subunit is important. Gentle handling of the tissue and minimal use of cautery limit the tissues inflammatory response during the early wound-healing phase. Undermining of the surgical site should be completed to allow for minimal tension at the site of closure. Appropriate suture selection can help minimize the inflammatory response. Resorbable sutures that degrade as a result of hydrolysis, such as Monocryl Suture, as opposed to those that resorb as a result of inflammatory mediators should be considered. When approximating the epidermis, suture materials, such as prolene and nylon, should be considered and removed between day 5 and day 7. At the time of closure, the wound can be bathed with triamcinolone and in select areas within the head and neck, such as the forehead and neck, chemodenervation with botulinum toxin can be placed to minimized muscular tension on the wound and thus minimize fibroblast proliferation.[2]

Postsurgical treatment should be implemented to minimize inflammation, proliferation, and wound contraction. The early use of oral antihistamines and intralesional triamcinolone can help decrease inflammatory mediators during early wound healing. The topical application of immunomodulators, such as imiquimod, can help decrease fibroblast proliferation and the use of silicone sheeting or occlusive dressings can assist with long-term healing and wound remodeling.[1]

Against this backdrop, when treating suspected keloid formers, multimodality long-term follow-up is essential to minimize the development of keloids or hyptertrophic scars.

BOAHENE

Prior to surgical resection of keloids in a known keloid former, I pretreat the surgical bed with triamcinolone. I inject triamcinolone in the normal tissue just adjacent to the keloid tissue and not the keloid mass. My rationale is to target fibroblast in the normal dermis, which is activated to heal the final incisional scar. I inject 3 times, 6 weeks to 8 weeks apart, prior to surgery. When my surgical goal is to reduce the size of the keloid rather than completely resect it, then I limit the triamcinolone injection to the keloid scar. To facilitate ease and spread of the triamcinolone, I occasionally inject collagenase into the keloid days before the steroid injection. I have not formally studied the combined effect of collagenase and triamcinolone but have patient feedback of less pain during injection.

JONES

My prophylactic protocol for treating keloids begins with the initial consultation. I ask patients what outcomes are important. I have found that patients are often looking for relief of symptoms, such as itching, pain, frequent infections, foul drainage, and loss of function. Others are concerned about cosmesis. I usually explain that all their concerns may not be addressed and, if it is possible to remove the keloid and eliminate all symptoms, there is an unknown risk of recurrence and the keloid and symptoms may return and be worse than if no treatment were attempted. I also, explain why it is okay to forgo therapy. Patients must weigh the risk and benefit of treatment. If therapy is chosen, I try to tailor it to the individual patient. I then discuss a plan to manage confounding conditions, such as referral to dermatology for acne treatment, plan for laser hair removal, discontinuation of wearing earrings, antibiotics and wound care regimen for recurrent infections, and supportive garments to eliminate tension on the keloid site. Treatment of pain and itching is also important to prevent irritation of the treatment area from frequent scratching and rubbing. Patients have to be willing to commit to a long-term treatment plan with close follow-up prior to starting a treatment regimen.

Question 4: How long do you treat or follow patients after surgical removal?

BRISSETT

When considering the treatment duration for patients with keloids, it is important to recognize that this disease process represents a chronic illness with high recurrence rates, without definitive cure, and with unpredictable duration times for recurrence.[1–3]

Educating patients on the nuances of this disease process is critical when defining their follow-up strategy, thus minimizing the likelihood of recurrence. The estimated duration of keloid recurrence can vary anywhere from 3 months to several years. A majority of recurrences begin to manifest themselves within the first year of treatment. There is a constellation of signs and symptoms that herald the onset of keloid recurrence, such as firmness and redness of the scar or surrounding tissue and itching or discomfort.[5]

The postsurgical treatment of keloids and hypertrophic scars is focused on limiting the signs and symptoms of recurrence and reactivation in addition to minimizing the development of proliferative tissue. If keloid regrowth does occur, treatment is then focused on preventing further growth.

Against this background, patient education and long-term follow-up are required for the successful management of the patient suffering from keloids. The postsurgical treatment protocol should be focused on eliminating signs of early recurrence and addressing symptoms of reactivation. As with any chronic disease, the duration of follow-up is indeterminate and ongoing. Close and frequent follow-up is required for the first year. At that point follow-up can be quarterly, biannually, or annually. It is important that patients are educated to recognize early signs of reactivation and recurrence and present to their surgeon in a timely manner for treatment to minimize regrowth.

JONES

I believe patients should be followed for a minimum of 1 year after treatment of keloids. Surgical treatment is always associated with dual or multimodality therapy. Most patients have a treatment protocol requiring frequent visits, which are spread out over several weeks or months. The length of treatment varies with adjuvant therapy. Postsurgical triamcinolone and/or 5-FU injections are done every 4 weeks to 6 weeks for up to a year. Pressure therapy, such as pressure earrings after keloid removal, must be maintained for at least a year. Laser therapy for hair removal is performed every several weeks until satisfactory hair reduction is obtained. I explain that they should be watchful and not be complacent because there are no signs of recurrence in the initial posttherapy period. I educate patients on signs of keloid recurrence and associated symptoms. They are encouraged to seek prompt evaluation for suspected recurrences.

BOAHENE

I typically follow patients who have responded to surgical treatment for at least 1 year. I inject the resection bed 3 times at 6-week to 8-week intervals with triamcinolone. After the regimen of steroid injection, I see patients back every 3 months through the first postoperative year. I instruct patients to return for follow-up should there be any signs of recurrence or progression of keloid activity. Increased itching commonly heralds keloid activity. I counsel patients to avoid repiercing their ears if that was the cause of their keloids. I emphasize that keloids are not cured but controlled. Long-term follow-up is, therefore, necessary but patient directed.

Question 5: When do you consider radiation therapy for the management of keloids?

BOAHENE

For more than a century, radiation therapy has been used to treat keloids. The treatment of a benign disease with radiotherapy, however, is not without controversy given historic experience with secondary malignancies. It is generally accepted that surgery as a single-modality treatment of keloids is associated with a high recurrence rate. As such, many centers combine surgery with other modalities, such as intralesional injection of triamcinolone or 5-FU and postsurgical radiotherapy. There are no clear indications for the use of postsurgical radiotherapy in the treatment of keloids. I consider radiation therapy for resistant keloids. Resistant keloids are refractory scars that have failed multiple levels of conventional treatment and recurrences that threaten adjacent functional structures, such as the ear canal. The number of failed treatments that trigger my recommendation for radiation therapy depends on the location of the keloid, risk to adjacent structures, rapidity and extent of recurrence, and thoroughness and response to previous treatment regimen.

Two main factors should be considered when recommending radiation for keloids: safety and effectiveness. The main safety concern with using radiation is the potential for secondary malignancies arising in the treatment field. A review of the literature from 1901 when radiographs were used to the contemporary treatment with external-beam therapy concludes that the risk of secondary malignancies is extremely low. In an exhaustive literature review, Ogawa and colleagues[1] found only 5 reported cases of radiation-induced malignancies after keloid treatment. With proper dosing and planning, the risk for secondary malignancies resulting from radiation treatment of keloids is extremely low.

The effectiveness of postsurgical radiotherapy in controlling keloids seems dose dependent.

It is recommended that a biologic effective dose of at least 30 Gy be given. Radiation therapy should be initiated within 48 hours of surgical resection. Patients should be counseled about the potential for the usual adverse effects of radiation therapy, including acute skin reactions and persistent pigmentary changes.

The technique for administering postsurgical radiation to keloids has evolved over the years, transitioning from radiographs to electron beams and more recently brachytherapy with iridium Ir 192. Brachytherapy allows for a more tailored and concentrated irradiation of the targeted bed while sparing normal tissues.

BRISSETT

I consider the use of radiation therapy on patients who have a history of recurrent keloids recalcitrant to standard treatment protocols, such as injectable therapy, surgery, and immunomodulators. In general, I reserve the use of radiation therapy for patients that have failed traditional treatment protocols.

JONES

I consider radiation for recurrent keloids. I also consider radiation as adjuvant therapy for large areas that require reconstruction with skin grafts or local flaps. I believe that radiation therapy, which is usually over 12 Gy, also treats acne and causes hair loss, frequent contributors to keloid formation in the beard, scalp, and cheek areas. Patients should be counseled in advance about the potential long-term risk of radiation therapy, including a remote risk of cancer and the likelihood of alopecia because doses over 7 Gy cause permanent hair loss.

Question 6: What is your prophylactic protocol when operating on known keloid formers?

BOAHENE

There are several patient-related factors that increase the risk of forming keloids after surgery. These include a known history of previous keloid formation, familial aggregation of keloid scarring, a twin with a history of keloids, and Asian or African ancestry. When elective surgery is planned in such high-risk patients, proactive measures before, during, and after the procedure may be taken to minimize the risk of keloid formation.

Whenever possible, surgical approaches that avoid external skin incisions should be considered. For example, a submandibular gland resection may be performed transorally through a vestibular mucosal incision to avoid an external neck incision and a robotic-assisted transoral thyroidectomy may be considered over an open transcervical approach. External skin incisions, when unavoidable, should be minimized and visualization of the surgical bed enhanced with endoscopic visualizations.

When operating in a surgical bed with previous keloid, steroid may be injected around the keloid scar weeks prior to the planned elective surgery. I usually inject the normal skin around the keloid with triamcinolone 3 weeks to 6 weeks prior to the scheduled procedure. Steroids may also be injected at the time of surgery.

Koloids are frequently observed in wounds experiencing high tensile forces.

Techniques that minimize tension of the final wound are helpful. These include the use of deep tension retaining sutures and external supportive taping. Immobilizing muscles around the wound that can distract the suture line with botulinum injection has been shown to improve scarring on the forehead. The main goal of chemoimmobilization of cutaneous wounds is to eliminate dynamic tension on the healing tissues. Paralysis of the muscle groups adjacent and subjacent to the wound should, therefore, be as complete as possible. Beyond the forehead, chemoimmobilization may apply in other surgical sites where direct muscle action may pull on the final wound.

To minimize scarring and suture track marks, subcuticular closure, early removal of skin sutures, and the use of tissue adhesives should be considered. In high-risk keloid formers, early application of topical silicone gel sheeting has been shown useful in the preventing hypertrophic scars and keloids in patients undergoing scar revision. Silicone application may be initiated within 48 hours of wound closure.

Despite these measures, hypertrophic scarring and keloids may still occur and close follow-up is necessary. Intralesional steroid injection performed early may arrest and reverse the progression of undesirable scarring.

JONES

I believe surgery, in many cases, is the only way to completely remove the keloid and associated symptoms. I explain, however, that surgery should never be used as a single modality to treat keloids and should always be combined with other adjuvant therapies, such as topical or injection of steroids, injectable 5-FU, radiation, and the application of pressure therapy. I believe incisions should be limited and placed in relaxed skin tension lines and at the junction of aesthetic units, whenever possible. I try to limit wound closure tension and use deep sutures, whenever possible, to reduce tension on the skin closure. I avoid absorbable sutures for the skin. When using permanent sutures for skin closure, I either use a subcuticular technique or remove running sutures in 5 days, whenever possible.

BRISSETT

There are several patient-related factors that increase the risk of forming keloids after surgery. These include a known history of previous keloid formation, familial aggregation of keloid scarring, a twin with a history of keloids, and Asian or African ancestry. When elective surgery is planned in such high-risk patients, proactive measures before, during, and after the procedure may be taken to minimize the risk of keloid formation.

Whenever possible, surgical approaches that avoid external skin incisions should be considered. For example, a submandibular gland resection may be performed transorally through a vestibular mucosal incision to avoid an external neck incision and a robotic-assisted transoral thyroidectomy may be considered over an open transcervical approach. External skin incisions, when unavoidable, should be minimized and visualization of the surgical bed enhanced with endoscopic visualizations.

When operating in a surgical bed with previous keloid, steroid may be injected around the keloid scar weeks prior to the planned elective surgery. I usually inject the normal skin around the keloid with triamcinolone 3 weeks to 6 weeks prior to the scheduled procedure. Steroids may also be injected at the time of surgery.

Keloids are frequently observed in wounds experiencing high tensile forces.

Techniques that minimize tension of the final wound are helpful. These include the use of deep tension retaining sutures and external supportive taping. Immobilizing muscles around the wound that can distract the suture line with botulinum injection has been shown to improve scarring on the forehead. The main goal of chemoimmobilization of cutaneous wounds is to eliminate dynamic tension on the healing tissues. Paralysis of the muscle groups adjacent and subjacent to the wound should, therefore, be as complete as possible. Beyond the forehead, chemoimmobilization may apply in other surgical sites where direct muscle action may pull on the final wound.

To minimize scarring and suture track marks, subcuticular closure, early removal of skin sutures, and the use of tissue adhesives should be considered. In high-risk keloid formers, early application of topical silicone gel sheeting has been shown useful in the preventing hypertrophic scars and keloids in patients undergoing scar revision. Silicone application may be initiated within 48 hours of wound closure.

Despite these measures, hypertrophic scarring and keloids may still occur and close follow-up is necessary. Intralesional steroid injection performed early may arrest and reverse the progression of undesirable scarring.

REFERENCES

1. Ogawa R, Yoshitatsu S, Yoshida K, et al. Is radiation therapy for keloids acceptable? The risk of radiation-induced carcinogenesis. Plast Reconstr Surg 2009; 124(4):1196–201.
2. Xu J, Yang E, Yu NZ, et al. Radiation therapy in keloids treatment: history, strategy, effectiveness, and complication. Chin Med J (Engl) 2017;130(14): 1715–21.
3. Kelly AP. Medical and surgical therapies for keloids. Dermatol Ther 2004;17:212–8.
4. Mustoe TA, Cooter RD, Gold MH, et al. International clinical recommendations on scar management. Plast Reconstr Surg 2002;110:560–71.
5. Brody GS. Keloids and hypertrophic scars. Plast Reconstr Surg 1990;86:804.
6. Careta MF, Fortes AC, Messina MC, et al. Combined treatment of earlobe keloids with shaving, cryosurgery, and intralesional steroid injection: a 1-year follow-up. Dermatol Surg 2013;39(5):734–8.
7. Guy WM, Pattisapu P, Ongkasuwan J, et al. Creation of a head and neck Keloid quality of life questionnaire. Laryngoscope 2015;125(12):2672–6.
8. Naylor MC, Brissett AE. Current concepts in the etiology and treatment of keloids. Facial Plast Surg 2012;28(5):504–12.
9. Gassner HG, Brissett AE, Otley CC, et al. Botulinum toxin to improve facial wound healing: a prospective, blinded, placebo-controlled study. Mayo Clin Proc 2006;81(8):1023–8.
10. Gold MH, Foster TD, Adair MA, et al. Prevention of hypertrophic scars and keloids by the prophylactic use of topical silicone gel sheets following a surgical procedure in an office setting. Dermatol Surg 2001; 27(7):641–4.
11. Jones LR, Greene J, Chen KM, et al. Biological significance of genome-wide DNA methylation profiles in keloids. Laryngoscope 2017;127(1):70–8.
12. Fujiwara M, Muragaki Y, Ooshima A. Keloid-derived fibroblasts show increased secretion of factors involved in collagen turnover and depend on matrix

metalloproteinase for migration. Br J Dermatol 2005; 153:295–300.

13. Hahn JM, Glaser K, McFarland KL, et al. Keloid-derived keratinocytes exhibit an abnormal gene expression profile consistent with a distinct causal role in keloid pathology. Wound Repair Regen 2013;21:530–44.

14. Jumper N, Hodgkinson T, Paus R, et al. Site-specific gene expression profiling as a novel strategy for unravelling keloid disease pathobiology. PLoS One 2017;12:e0172955.

15. Funayama E, Chodon T, Oyama A, et al. Keratinocytes promote proliferation and inhibit apoptosis of the underlying fibroblasts: an important role in the pathogenesis of keloid. J Invest Dermatol 2003; 121:1326 31.

16. He Y, Deng Z, Alghamdi M, et al. From genetics to epigenetics: new insights into keloid scarring. Cell Prolif 2017;50(2):e12326.

17. Shih B, Garside E, McGrouther DA, et al. Molecular dissection of abnormal wound healing processes resulting in keloid disease. Wound Repair Regen 2010;18:139–53.

FURTHER READINGS

Alexis A, Heath CR, Halder RM. Folliculitis keloidalis nuchae and pseudofolliculitis barbae: are prevention and effective treatment within reach? Dermatol Clin 2014;32:183–91.

Bran GM, Goessler UR, Hormann K, et al. Keloids: current concepts of pathogenesis (review). Int J Mol Med 2009;24:283–93.

Butler PD, Longaker MT, Yang GP. Current progress in keloid research and treatment. J Am Coll Surgeons 2008;206:731–41.

Davis SA, Feldman SR, McMichael AJ. Management of keloids in the United States, 1990-2009: an analysis of the National Ambulatory Medical Care Survey. Dermatol Surg 2013;39:988–94.

He S, Liu X, Yang Y, et al. Mechanisms of transforming growth factor beta(1)/Smad signalling mediated by mitogen-activated protein kinase pathways in keloid fibroblasts. Br J Dermatol 2010;162:538–46.

Jones LR, Young W, Divine G, et al. Genome-wide scan for methylation profiles in keloids. Dis markers 2015; 2015:943176.

Kelly AP. Pseudofolliculitis barbae and acne keloidalis nuchae. Dermatol Clin 2003;21:645–53.

Lane JE, Waller JL, Davis LS. Relationship between age of ear piercing and keloid formation. Pediatrics 2005;115:1312–4.

Marttala J, Andrews JP, Rosenbloom J, et al. Keloids: animal models and pathologic equivalents to study tissue fibrosis. Matrix Biol 2016;51:47–54.

Muir IF. On the nature of keloid and hypertrophic scars. Br J Plast Surg 1990;43:61–9.

Satish L, Babu M, Tran KT, et al. Keloid fibroblast responsiveness to epidermal growth factor and activation of downstream intracellular signaling pathways. Wound Repair Regen 2004;12:183–92.

Shih B, Bayat A. Genetics of keloid scarring. Arch Dermatol Res 2010;302:319–39.

Strimbu K, Tavel JA. What are biomarkers? Curr Opin HIV AIDS 2010;5:463–6.

Tuan TL, Nichter LS. The molecular basis of keloid and hypertrophic scar formation. Mol Med Today 1998; 4:19–24.

van den Broek LJ, Limandjaja GC, Niessen FB, et al. Human hypertrophic and keloid scar models: principles, limitations and future challenges from a tissue engineering perspective. Exp Dermatol 2014;23:382–6.

Young WG, Worsham MJ, Joseph CL, et al. Incidence of keloid and risk factors following head and neck surgery. JAMA Facial Plast Surg 2014;16(5):379–80.

Contemporary Laser and Light-Based Rejuvenation Techniques

Mark Hamilton, MD[a],*, Andrew Campbell, MD[b],
J. David Holcomb, MD[c]

KEYWORDS

- Laser resurfacing • Fractional laser resurfacing • Erbium:YAG laser • CO_2 laser • Hybrid fractional
- Photoaging • Rhytids • Ablative

KEY POINTS

- The main wavelengths used for skin rejuvenation continue to be the CO_2 and the erbium:YAG. Improvements in devices include fractional technology, combination with other wavelengths, and deeper penetrating spot sizes.
- Whether CO_2 or erbium, full-field resurfacing remains the technique of choice for those Fitzpatrick types 1 and 2 patients with deep rhytids and extensive photodamage.
- For younger patients with an active lifestyle, fractional and hybrid devices offer new opportunities for skin rejuvenation with minimal downtime and minimal risks.
- Laser skin rejuvenation in darker skin types remains a challenge, although newer devices offer the possibility of safe treatment.
- The overall laser skin rejuvenation field has grown tremendously with fractional and hybrid devices, creating most of this expansion.

Question 1: What is your choice of device for extreme sun damage and aged skin (Glogau 4) in Fitzpatrick types 1, 2 and why? Give typical settings?

HAMILTON

For those patients with extensive photodamage and deep wrinkles who are done with the sun and desire maximal improvement, full-field CO_2 laser resurfacing is the best option. This technique has a proven track record of consistent, effective results. The simplicity and speed of these treatments are far superior to erbium techniques. It has been listed as the gold standard for maximal facial rejuvenation, and I believe that has not changed.[1]

Although CO_2 laser does produce more heat deposition, this provides an advantage, especially in more severe cases. Depositing heat causes collagen and thus tissue contraction. This provides further skin tightening as well as wrinkle reduction. In cases needing consistent maximal wrinkle reduction, only CO_2 laser is able to provide this.

Although deep penetrating fractional lasers offer an interesting alternative for deep rhytids, the results for the most part have been disappointing. Despite the ability to offer much deeper depths of penetration, the decrease in skin surface area

---

Disclosure Statement: M. Hamilton is on the Speakers Bureau for Allergan. A. Campbell and J.D. Holcomb have nothing to disclose.
[a] Hamilton Facial Plastic Surgery, 533 East County Line Road, Suite #104, Greenwood, IN 46143, USA;
[b] Quintessa Aesthetic Centers, 2124 Kohler Memorial Drive, Sheboygan, WI 53081, USA; [c] Holcomb-Kreithen Plastic Surgery, 1 South School Avenue, Suite 800, Sarasota, FL 34237, USA
* Corresponding author.
E-mail address: mhamilton@hamiltonfps.com

Facial Plast Surg Clin N Am 26 (2018) 113–121
https://doi.org/10.1016/j.fsc.2017.12.002

Panel Discussion

1. What is your choice of device for extreme sun damage and aged skin (Glogau 4) in Fitzpatrick types 1, 2 and why? Give typical settings.

2. How do you approach patients who need surgical lifting as well as skin resurfacing?

3. What is your choice for rejuvenation of skin in higher Fitzpatrick skin types (3–6)? Typical settings?

4. How do you approach the young patient with early aging (Glogau 1, 2)?

5. What techniques do you use to speed along post–laser healing?

6. How have your techniques with laser and light-based facial rejuvenation changed in the last 5 years?

covered has precluded comparable wrinkle improvement to full-field resurfacing in a single session. Even with multiple treatments, maximal improvement in difficult cases with fractional devices just cannot match full-field resurfacing.

For laser resurfacing, I use the Lumenis Encore. This device is reliable and effective. Procedures are quick and bloodless. Typical settings vary depending on the patient as well as the device. That said, for extensive photodamage, settings of 100 to 125 mJ and a density of 5 are typically used. On average, 2 passes are made and possibly a third or fourth in more challenging cases. Passes after the second are typically done at a lower setting and only to select deep rhytids (**Fig. 1**).

CAMPBELL

I prefer the erbium:YAG laser by Sciton. The erbium laser is the most efficient way to ablate the skin because of its absorption spectrum. At 2940 nm, the laser only penetrates the skin about 4 μm, thus causing virtually all of the energy to be converted instantly to heat, vaporizing the skin. Because of this efficient absorption, there is very little heat transfer, limiting necrosis and heat shock of deeper tissue. This has been proven to greatly reduce the risk of hypopigmentation, hyperpigmentation, and prolonged healing. The duration and intensity of erythema are also greatly reduced, yet the wrinkle reduction has been shown to be equivalent to a CO_2 laser.[2] Basically, it gives me all of the benefits of the best wrinkle reduction while minimizing the side effects of hypopigmentation, hyperpigmentation, and erythema of the CO_2 laser.

For deep rhytids, the settings I use are typically 200 μm per pass at 50% overlap. One to 3 passes are made across most areas of the face, but the perioral region can be treated with up to 8 passes (my personal maximum; most patients are treated with 3–4 passes) as needed. The periorbital area is treated with 80 μm with 25 μm of coagulation. This treatment of the periorbital area seems to help tighten the thinner periorbital skin safely when making 2 to 3 passes. The passes are tapered across the jawline. The neck can safely be treated with 25 to 80 μm.

HOLCOMB

Dual-mode erbium-YAG laser and fractional CO_2 laser are used in combination. This approach conserves the benefits of full-field deep laser skin resurfacing while also incorporating the benefits of ablative fractional resurfacing. Patients that have significant to extreme skin photoaging typically have significant dyschromia and deep rhytids and may have actinic changes. Full-field ablative laser skin resurfacing with the erbium-YAG laser will substantially resolve surface concerns with a single pass of adequate depth (dual-mode erbium-YAG; eg, 100-200 ablate, 0 coagulate, 50% overlap, 4-mm spot). Treatment with the fractional CO_2 laser immediately follows to further the goals of rhytid reduction and skin tightening (eg, 120-μm spot, 55 mJ, 15% surface area coverage). For the most severe rhytids, additional passes with the erbium-YAG laser and/or use of a larger spot size and higher energy and coverage with the fractional CO_2 laser (eg, 1000 μm, 200 mJ, 100% surface area coverage) may occasionally be warranted (**Fig. 2**).

Question 2: How do you approach patients who need surgical lifting as well as skin resurfacing?

HAMILTON

Multiple studies have shown that CO_2 laser resurfacing can be safely combined with a facelift.[3] Important factors in making this combination safe include facelift technique and laser settings. The deep plane facelift offers a greater degree of safety for combined procedures. I use an extended SMAS biplanar facelift with a fair amount of skin undermining in some cases. It is important to lower the setting over areas of elevated skin. Fortunately, these are typically areas of less sun damage and wrinkling. For most cases, just one pass at a setting of 60 mJ or less and a density of 5 is made over the elevated tissues.

Fractional resurfacing provides an even greater margin of safety. Many patients undergoing

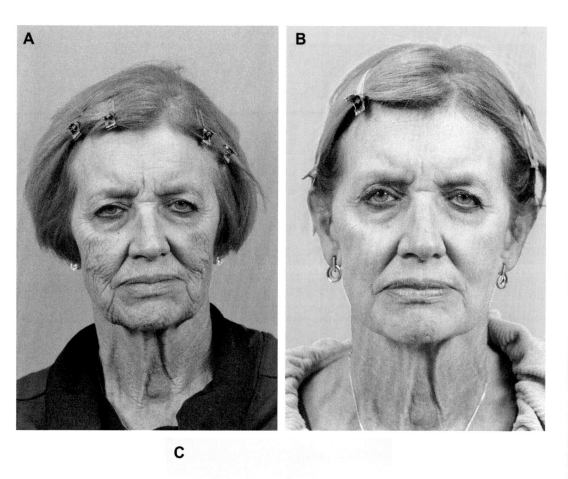

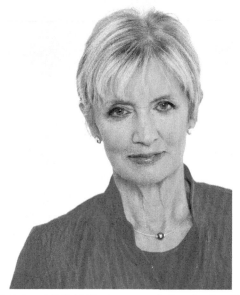

Fig. 1. Before (*A*) and after (*B*) full-face full-field CO_2 laser resurfacing. Setting: Two passes were made at 100 mJ, density of 5; a second and third pass were made to select rhytids. The periorbital area was treated at a fluence of 80 mJ and density of 4. Note hypopigmentation after laser. (*C*) With makeup.

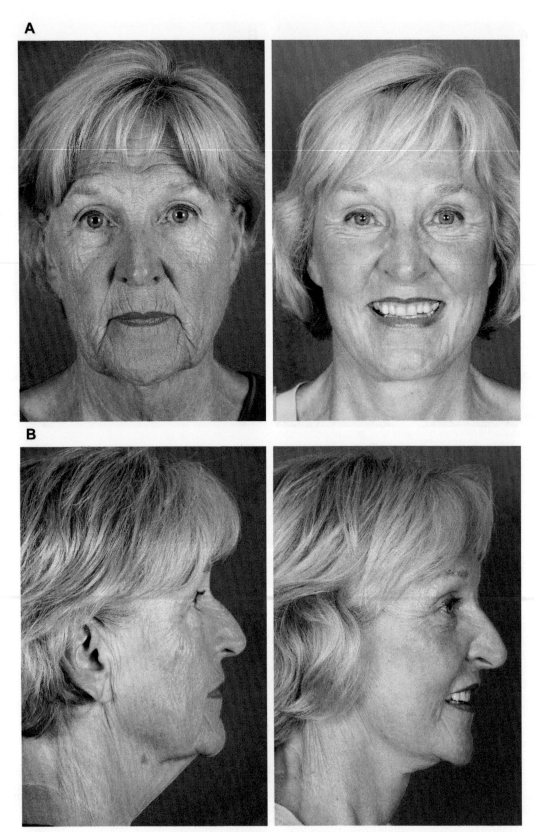

Fig. 2. Before and after facelift with full-face erbium laser resurfacing. (*A*) Front view. (*B*) Side view.

simultaneous rhytidectomy with resurfacing do not need as aggressive laser treatment. Fractional laser resurfacing offers a nice alternative with surprisingly good results when combined with lifting. I still typically use a lower setting over elevated tissues than elsewhere and never use the deep fractional settings in these areas.

In addition, resurfacing can be safely combined with blepharoplasty and forehead lift procedures. As with rhytidectomy, fractional settings may be used with an even greater level of safety and a quicker recovery.

CAMPBELL

I approach patients that need both surgical lifting and skin resurfacing with confidence. I personally perform high SMAS deep plane facelifts, which create a thick and very well-vascularized facelift flap. When elevating and fixating the deep plane, there is only about 1 cm of subcutaneous flap that is left. I therefore routinely perform deep laser resurfacing on my facelift patients without concern for necrosis. I will taper the depth directly in front of the ear to under 100 μm, but otherwise treat the facial skin as I would had I not performed a facelift with the laser resurfacing. I have yet to see any necrosis related to the combination of laser resurfacing with the facelift. If I was doing a standard subcutaneous/SMAS lift, I would limit the resurfacing to 80 μm or less on any skin that has undergone immediate subcutaneous elevation.

HOLCOMB

Concurrent facial surgery and skin resurfacing is safe and commonly performed. The concern for maintaining surgical flap viability is paramount. The surgical approach does have bearing on the treatment settings for photodamaged skin over undermined areas of the surgical flap. Although deep plane facelift flaps should tolerate more aggressive laser skin resurfacing settings than cutaneous facelift flaps, it is generally the case that the skin over the posterior aspect of the cheek is less affected by rhytidosis than in other areas of the face. My surgical facelift approach involves a multiplanar approach with variable length cutaneous skin flaps; therefore, I limit laser treatment settings in this area (eg, 50 μm laser skin peel with dual-mode erbium-YAG laser *or* 10% coverage with 120-μm spot at 40–55 mJ with fractional CO_2 laser) compared with the cheek skin anterior to the extent of surgical undermining.

Question 3: What is your choice for rejuvenation of skin in higher Fitzpatrick skin types (3–6)? Typical settings?

HAMILTON

Laser resurfacing in darker skin types continues to be a challenge. Fractional CO_2 laser may be used in many patients who would not be candidates for full-field laser resurfacing. Even so, concerns for hyperpigmentation remain high. Typically, settings are lower, and pretreatment with bleaching agents may be advised. Fortunately, these patients typically have less need for aggressive laser techniques because of less wrinkling and sun damage. A setting of 80 mJ and a density of 1 provide some improvement with a degree of safety.

The Fraxel 1550-nm device offers the ability to safely treat all skin types. It has been particularly helpful with resurfacing for acne scarring. Multiple treatments are required.

Our own experience has been mixed, but this does offer a safe option for these challenging cases. Microneedling is another non-light-based treatment that may offer the best option and an inexpensive one at that. It is presently our first choice for improving rhytids, texture, and acne scarring in darker skin types.

CAMPBELL

For patients with darker skin, I prefer the Halo laser. This laser is a hybrid fractional laser incorporating a 1470-nm nonablative laser with the 2940-nm erbium laser. The lasers work synergistically to create significant dermal neocollagenesis, wrinkle reduction, and skin tightening. We have used this laser on skin types up to 5 without hyperpigmentation, although we did see some post–inflammatory hyperpigmentation on a skin type 3 when very deep settings were used. Our typical settings are 400 μm, 1470 nm with 20 to 40 μm erbium at 20% density. We will treat deeper rhytids at 30% to 40% density with the same depths. With these settings, we have not seen any hyperpigmentation, hypopigmentation, or scarring in any patient, yet we can get pretty remarkable improvement in pigmentation, vascularity, texture, wrinkles, and even the appearance of pores. For skin type 6, I have no personal experience, but would test spot the Halo with the settings of 400 μm, 1470 nm and 20 μm erbium at 20%. I would expect to see no problems.

HOLCOMB

Postprocedure dyschromias (including high incidence of PIH or post–inflammatory hyperpigmentation and a much lower incidence of hypopigmentation) are of increasing concern with increasing Fitzpatrick Skin Type score. In addition, the typical concerns of moderate to severe rhytidosis and mild dyschromia seen in lighter Fitzpatrick Skin types (eg I, II) are often replaced with concerns of refractory dark pigmentation and only mild rhytidosis in darker Fitzpatrick Skin types (eg III, IV, V, VI).

Although ablative laser therapy (both full field and ablative fractional resurfacing [AFR]) may be highly beneficial for the former group, even conservative AFR may be problematic for the latter group with high likelihood of PIH. Patients with the intermediate Fitzpatrick Skin type III may be treated with satisfactory outcomes with either full-field ablative laser skin resurfacing or AFR.

Development of PIH increases with density of ablative coverage (full field > fractionated) and with severity of inflammatory response to ablative treatment (CO_2 > erbium-YAG). Nonablative fractional laser skin resurfacing (NFR) and treatment with the hybrid fractional laser (1470 NFR with microablative erbium-YAG 20- to 100-μm depth) are additional options for treatment of skin photoaging and dyschromia in darker skin types.

Question 4: How do you approach the young patient with early aging (Glogau 1, 2)?

HAMILTON

Fractional CO_2 laser resurfacing and intense pulsed light (IPL) are outstanding options for early aging in the young patient. For those with early wrinkling and photodamage, fractional technology provides an excellent option. Skin coloration is often improved with just one treatment. Wrinkle reduction usually requires multiple sessions and deeper penetrating technology. Patients can have multiple treatments over time with virtually no risk of color loss. In addition, treatments can often be done in the office with just topical anesthesia and dental blocks. Downtime is typically 4 to 6 days with almost all patients able to wear makeup by 1 week. Redness may persist for 2 to 4 weeks and rarely beyond this. Although fractional technology does not provide the same degree of correction as full-field resurfacing, for those who have an active life, continue to be in the sun, and are accepting of more subtle changes, it provides a great option (**Fig. 3**).

IPL remains an undervalued and relatively inexpensive technology. Although providing excellent correction of reds and browns, it also provides a surprisingly nice improvement in the tone and luminescence of skin. With multiple treatments, one may even see a subtle improvement in fine lines. These results are often comparable to those achieved with nonablative/combined devices, some of which have become extremely expensive.

CAMPBELL

A Halo laser is perfect for the younger patient with mild skin aging. The epidermis is healed within 24 hours, so patients can wear makeup the next day. Heavy moisturizer prevents the appearance of microscopic epidermal necrotic debris (MENDs), small flakes of skin that appear during healing. The MENDs are slightly darker than the surrounding skin, and this can be easily camouflaged with mineral makeup, so most patients go back to work the day after the treatment. Because of the synergy of the 2 lasers, the improvement in texture, pigment, vascularity, and wrinkles is impressive, especially considering the lack of downtime (**Fig. 4**).

HOLCOMB

Conservative laser treatments are ideal for younger patients with no wrinkles at rest and mild photodamage and dyschromia. Superficial erbium-YAG "mini" laser peels (eg, single pass at 100 to 200-μm ablate, 0–50 coagulate) are full-field therapeutic treatments that provide a healthy skin glow after a short recovery period of 4 to 7 days. "Light" CO_2 AFR treatments (eg, 120-μm spot, 40–55 mJ, 10% to 15% coverage) enable significant improvement and greater skin tightening but require a little more downtime (5–10 days). In addition, treatment with the Hybrid Fractional Laser (1470 NFR with microablative erbium-YAG) is a popular option with either no downtime or up to 1 day of downtime with a more aggressive treatment.

Question 5: What techniques do you use to speed along post–laser healing?

HAMILTON

For those patients undergoing full-field CO_2 laser resurfacing, Silon-TSR Face Mask (Biomed Sciences, Allentown, PA, USA) dressings show a remarkable ability to speed along the process. This semiocclusive dressing provides decreased discomfort and significantly increased healing. The dressing's benefits can be seen after just a couple of days with obvious demarcations of healing and redness between those areas covered with the dressing and those not covered with the dressing. Typically, we leave the dressing on for 3 days. Although patients are always happy to have the dressing removed at day 3, they have noticeably less discomfort and quicker healing compared with those who do not receive the dressing.

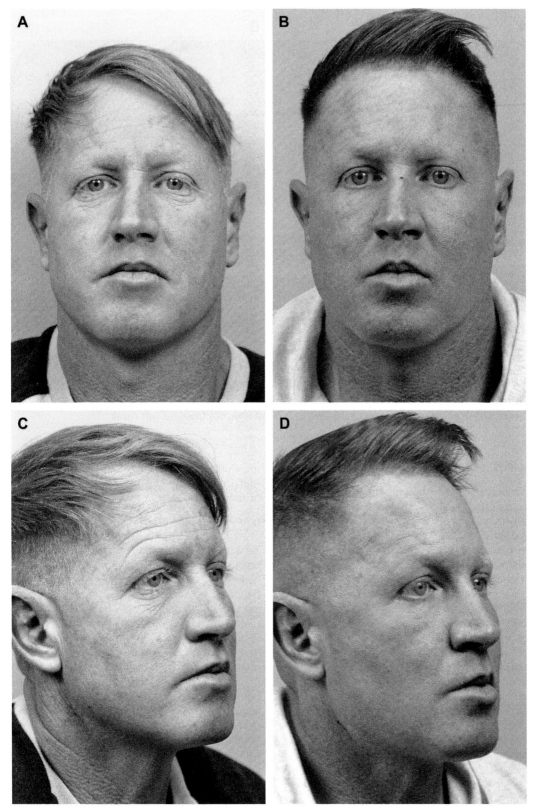

Fig. 3. Before (*A, C*) and after (*B, D*) full-face fractional CO_2 laser resurfacing. Deep FX was performed to the forehead and select rhytids at 17.5 to 20 mJ and a density of 5%. Active FX was performed to the entire face at 70 to 80 mJ and a density of 3.

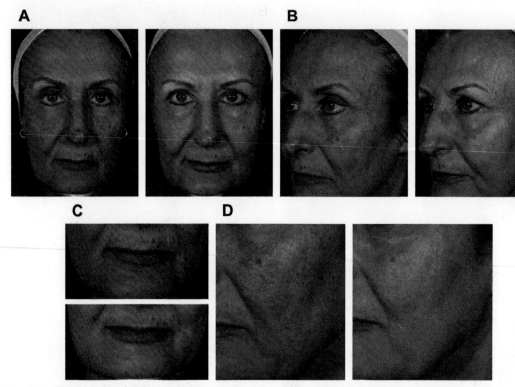

Fig. 4. Before and after full-face Halo laser treatment. Settings: single pass 20% treatment, 20 μm, 2940 and 400 μm, 1470. (*A*) Front view. (*B*) Left oblique view. (*C*) Perioral view. (*D*) Close-up, left cheek.

CAMPBELL

At Quintessa, for full-field erbium laser resurfacing, we use Bio2 Cosmeceutical's Oxy-Mist and Amino-Plex. Using compressed oxygen, Oxy-Mist is sprayed on the freshly lasered skin immediately after the resurfacing. Because the epidermis has been ablated, the dermis is exposed, and that is what the solution is sprayed on to and penetrates. Oxy-Mist has amino acids, nucleotides, vitamins, and minerals and helps the skin heal faster. Amino-Plex is the at-home variety of the product. The patient will cleanse the skin, apply Amino-Plex spray, and then apply the occlusive balm. This is repeated several times a day. Dilute vinegar soaks are also used to help break up the exudate that forms on the skin. The soaks also seem to help with itching and erythema. Almost all patients, even those that underwent an extremely deep full-field erbium laser resurfacing, are completely reepithelialized at 7 to 8 days. All patients are on 1 week of prophylactic antibiotics and antivirals, and a single-dose antifungal.

After a Halo laser, patients typically use a ceramide moisturizer and mineral makeup. Ceramide seems to be a strong enough moisturizer to prevent the appearance of the MENDs yet is very unlikely to cause any reaction or irritation.

HOLCOMB

Time to reepithelialization varies from patient to patient with similar treatments. I have tried a variety of adjunctive therapies (eg, platelet-rich plasma, perfluorodecalin oxygen emulsion, low-frequency ultrasound saline mist therapy, photobiomodulation therapy at 590 nm and 830 nm) to mitigate the time and severity of the initial healing period following ablative laser treatments. Although none of these provided any dramatic reduction in time to reepithelialization, I continue to use the low-frequency ultrasound saline mist therapy as part of our routine postlaser skin care regimen; patients find the treatment soothing and enjoyable, and both patients and clinical staff find it beneficial in helping to debride and cleanse the skin at various intervals (eg, posttreatment days, 1, 4, 7). Nouveau topical skin care therapy with antioxidants and peptides has significantly reduced the duration of postprocedure erythema for many of our patients.

Question 6: How have your techniques with laser and light-based facial rejuvenation changed in the last 5 years?

HAMILTON

I have noticed 3 major changes in my use of laser devices for facial rejuvenation in the last 5 years: less full-field resurfacing, increased fractional resurfacing, and a reawakening of the benefits of IPL (vs newer fractional and nonablative devices).

Although some patients still benefit and require full-field laser resurfacing, many opt for fractional resurfacing. With multiple treatments, they are able to achieve very good results even if not equal to full field. In the process, they are able to avoid the hypopigmentation associated with full-field carbon dioxide laser resurfacing, which is the number one concern and complaint. A key part of this change has been my recognition and patient acceptance that often they will need multiple treatment sessions with fractional resurfacing to achieve the results that they want, especially when it comes to wrinkle reduction.

Although increased use of fractional technology is in part from patients who may have had full field in the past, it is mostly due to just an increased number of patients in my practice undergoing resurfacing. Many patients who in years past may have had peels now opt for a fractional laser. There is also a great awareness of this technology. Primary reasons for this are its ability to help with rhytids and scarring (especially with the deeper penetrating technologies), the impression that it is more "state-of-the-art" (debatable), patient marketing, and predictability. I look at this also as just a part of the impressive growth overall in nonsurgical cosmetic procedures.

Last, I have referred more patients back for IPL, whose results surpass those of some of the newer, more expensive combination devices. I cannot tell you how often I attend a marketing session or course meeting wherein I see the results of newer combination devices and think "well, I could have achieved that with my IPL." It is important as we evaluate these newer and often pricy technologies to honestly compare results to well-proven devices that we already have. This will save both our patients and us a great deal of expense.

CAMPBELL

The biggest change that has occurred in my practice in the past 5 years is the decrease the in number of full-field erbium laser resurfacings that I perform. This procedure has 7 to 10 days of extreme downtime, mild risks, and weeks to months of time before the skin appears and feels normal. The positive aspects of full-field erbium resurfacing are that it can create intense wrinkle reduction and take the deepest of wrinkles, even extremely deep perioral rhytids, and virtually eliminate them safely and consistently. Because of the fact that the Halo laser can cause a very significant improvement in the pigmentation, vascularity, texture, and wrinkles in skin, all while essentially eliminating any downtime and risk, many of the patients I would have treated with a full-field erbium laser resurfacing are now treated with 1 or 2 (sometimes 3) Halo laser treatments. These treatments are performed in the office setting using topical anesthetic with essentially no risk. The results for mild to moderate rhytids are excellent, and therefore, only patients with severe rhytids are still treated with full-field erbium laser resurfacing.

HOLCOMB

In general, I would say that in many ways I have become a bit more conservative while focusing more on improved outcomes; where appropriate, relying on the benefits of combining erbium-YAG full-field ablative resurfacing with CO_2 AFR rather than more aggressive mono-laser-therapy treatments. The 1470- to 2940-nm hybrid fractional laser has become the "go-to" treatment of choice for mild to moderate photoaging and dyschromia. I have turned away from laser therapy in favor of a topical skin depigmentation treatment of patients of all skin types with refractory dyschromias.

REFERENCES

1. Ward D, Baker S. Long term results with carbon dioxide laser resurfacing of the face. Arch Facial Plast Surg 2008;10(4):238–43.

2. Khatri KA, Ross V, Grevelink JM, et al. Comparison of erbium:YAG and carbon dioxide lasers in resurfacing of facial rhytides. Arch Dermatol 1999;135:391–7.

3. Koch BB, Perkins SW. Simultaneous rhytidectomy and full face carbon dioxide laser resurfacing: a case series and meta-analysis. Arch Facial Plast Surg 2002;4(4):227–33.

Radiofrequency Technology in Face and Neck Rejuvenation

Richard D. Gentile, MD, MBA[a],*,
Brian M. Kinney, MD, MSME[b], Neil S. Sadick, MD[c]

KEYWORDS

- Skin tightening • Facial contouring • Radiofrequency • Microneedle radiofrequency
- Catheter-based radiofrequency • Monopolar • Bipolar • Multipolar

KEY POINTS

- It is important to select the best radiofrequency (RF) device type to ensure the best clinical outcome for the face and neck.
- RF device types can range from monopolar, bipolar, or multipolar to multi-generator.
- Thermal devices, such as RF, affect the tissues at the molecular level.
- It is the biochemical and bio-thermal processes' effect on soft tissues that produces an aesthetic improvement.

Panel discussion

1. What is your perception of how thermal devices, such as radiofrequency (RF), affect the tissues at the molecular level, ultimately resulting in the biochemical and bio-thermal processes' effect on soft tissues that constitute an aesthetic improvement?

2. Based on cellular death paradigms, how can we explain the effects that ultimately occur after exposure to RF because of the hyperthermal environment? Specifically, what role do pyroptosis (electroporation) and apoptosis play in addition to coagulative necrosis? Do you think fractional microneedle RF provides a level of mechanical poration of adipose cells in addition to electroporation of cell membranes.?

3. Monopolar, bipolar, multipolar, and multi-generator RF for the face and neck: How do you select the best RF device type to ensure the best clinical outcome?

4. Do you agree or disagree with the following: Using the same number of RF treatments and the same type of RF device in the face and neck guarantees homogeneous skin tightening effects?

5. What are the best ways to address tissue selectively in the face and neck with RF?

6. What temperatures are indicated for nerve ablation, tissue tightening, skin rejuvenation, and stimulating an inflammatory response?

7. How have you changed your use of energy-based technologies over the last 5 years?

Disclosure Statement: The authors have nothing to disclose.
[a] Gentile Facial Plastic and Aesthetic Laser Center, 821 Kentwood Suite C, Youngstown, OH 44512, USA; [b] Plastic and Reconstructive Surgery, University of Southern California (USC), 120 South Spalding Drive, Suite 330, Beverly Hills, CA 90212, USA; [c] Weill Cornell Medical College, 911 Park Avenue, New York, NY 10075, USA
* Corresponding author.
E-mail address: dr-gentile@msn.com

Question 1: What is your perception of how thermal devices, such as radiofrequency, affect the tissues at the molecular level, ultimately resulting in biochemical and bio-thermal processes' effect on soft tissues that constitute an aesthetic improvement?

GENTILE

Radiofrequency (RF) devices work differently from optical lasers and photo-modulation. When laser light is delivered to the skin, there is an associated upregulation of matrix metalloproteinases that leads to a cellular response in the dermal collagen of the skin occurring either via water and collagen absorption of the light leading to a thermal effect on the dermis or through the production of growth factors and cellular mediators as a result of the light energy interacting with the hemoglobin and melanin within the skin. It has been postulated that nonablative lasers cause an increase in the production of type I procollagen messenger RNA (mRNA) associated with the tissue response occurring within the dermal matrix.

RF energy, on the other hand, uses resistive heating within the various layers of the skin to transform the RF energy given to the skin into thermal energy.[1–3] Resistive heating is also described as dielectric heating in which a high-frequency alternating electric field with associated magnetic fields or radio wave or microwave electromagnetic radiation heats a dielectric (polar) material. At the molecular level though, the total charge on a molecule is zero; the nature of chemical bonds is such that the positive and negative charges do not completely overlap in most molecules. Such molecules are said to be polar because they possess a permanent dipole moment. A good example is the dipole moment of the water molecule (**Fig. 1**). At higher frequencies, this heating is caused by molecular dipole rotation within the dielectric polar molecule. When no electric field is present, the molecules are randomly oriented. When the field is turned on, the molecules tend to line up with their negative ends toward the positive pole and their positive ends toward the negative pole. The oscillation of polar molecules produces frictional heating, ultimately generating the thermal effects to adjacent tissues in the electromagnetic field.

Many considerations are required for there to be successful transfer of the RF energy into thermal energy, including the size and depth of the tissue being treated, as one needs to consider the tissue impedance of the skin being treated. Because RF energy produces an electrical current instead of a light source, tissue damage can be minimized and epidermal melanin is not damaged either. With this knowledge, RF energies can be used for patients of all skin types, that is, it is color blind and allows for different depths of penetration based on what is to be treated, allowing for ultimate collagen contraction and production of new collagen as well as elastin and hyaluronic acid.[4]

KINNEY

The basic mechanism of RF interaction with tissues is the induction of a current through charged molecules and ions in the intracellular and extracellular tissues. Several factors influence the electrical impedance, including hydration, extracellular water content and the presence of fat, muscle, protein, and nervous tissue. Each tissue conducts electricity variably

Molecular dipoles

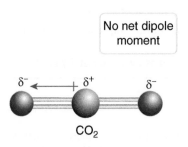

No net dipole moment

CO_2

The C=O bonds have dipoles of equal magnitude but opposite direction, so there is no net dipole moment.

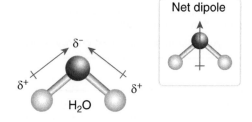

Net dipole

H_2O

The O–H bonds have dipoles of equal magnitude that do not cancel each other, so water has a net dipole moment.

Fig. 1. Dipole moment of the water molecule.

and has a different impedance (complex, time-varying resistance). Water is closest to a pure conductor. Fat is an insulator and has high resistance to current flow, thus, producing more heat during the flow of the induced electric field. The impedance increases in this order: water, nerves, muscles, collagen and other proteins, and finally fat. However, increasing order of tissue viability in the face of thermal heating is slightly different than for impedance and is shown in **Fig. 2**.

SADICK

Several studies have evaluated how RF affects the skin layers; molecular data point to a change in gene expression, including upregulation of heat shock proteins, cytokines (interleukin [IL]-1, IL-10) and growth factors (transforming growth factor β [TGF-β], vascular endothelial growth factor) that infiltrate the area. Histologic evidence also demonstrates that early after thermal stimulation there is partial or complete denaturation of the collagen fibril helix, collagen contraction, and dermal tissue swelling due to collagen injury. Long-term effects due to the activation of the wound healing cascade are increased expression of TGF-β, collagen and elastin remodeling, and reorientation, ultimately resulting in increased thickness of the papillary dermis. These molecular events both invigorate the area with growth factors and stimulate fibroblasts to produce collagen that rejuvenates and aesthetically improves the treated skin.[5–7]

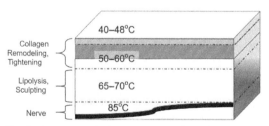

Fig. 2. Recommended temperatures for subcutaneous monopolar RF heating in the neck. Direct heat-induced contraction of collagen occurs within seconds at about 60°C, whereas stimulation of fibroblast in-migration and neocollagenesis is said to occur at about 47°C. Induction of adipocytolysis is thought to occur within 1 to 2 seconds at 70°C. Disabling of nerves with a fourth-degree injury (axonal, endoneurial, and perineurial disruption) lasting months is thought to occur within 1 minute at 85°C. (*Adapted from* Kinney BM, Andriessen A, DiBernardo BE, et al. Use of a controlled subdermal radio frequency thermistor for treating the aging neck: consensus recommendations. J Cosmet Laser Ther 2017;19(8):444–50; with permission.)

Question 2: Based on cellular death paradigms, how can we explain the effects that ultimately occur after exposure to radiofrequency because of the hyperthermal environment? Specifically, what role do pyroptosis (electroporation) and apoptosis play in addition to coagulative necrosis? Do you think fractional microneedle radiofrequency provides a level of mechanical poration of adipose cells in addition to electroporation of cell membranes?

GENTILE

Hyperthermic stimuli can elicit 2 distinct reactive cellular responses, the heat shock (stress) response and the activation of cell death pathways. Heat is a very effective means of killing tissue. As tissue temperature increases to greater than 113°F (50°C), protein is permanently damaged and cell membranes fuse. The process is rapid, typically requiring less than 10 to 15 minutes of exposure for a 3-cm ablation. In the cell death program, cells induce signaling pathways involving the coordinated action of multiple kinases and cysteine proteases, known as *caspases*, which cleave various target substrates, bringing about the cell's own demise.[8] This mode of programmed cell death is termed *apoptosis*, a genetically controlled suicide mechanism that does not produce an inflammatory response and is, therefore, considered a tidy method of cell elimination. Apoptosis is distinct from *necrosis*, which is a pathologic form of cell death in response to extreme trauma or environmental disruption. Morphologic alterations that are associated with necrosis include cell swelling, degeneration of organelles, membrane disruption, and cell lysis, causing inflammation.

Pyroptosis, discovered by Dr Brad Cookson, is a mechanism of cell death that exists in a space located somewhere between 2 polar opposites of apoptosis (silent, signaled cell death) and necrosis, often referred to as oncosis because of the invariable swelling response.[9] Pyroptosis exhibits some elements of both cell death pathways. The process of pyroptosis is mediated by caspase 1 and sometimes caspase 11. This process is called proinflammatory because secretion of both cytokines IL-1β and IL-8 are stimulated. Caspase 1 also causes poration of the cell membrane, with openings large enough to allow extracellular calcium inside the cell. Lysosomal and lipid droplets exit the cell, with depletion of cellular volume.[10]

Interestingly, in many patients treated with fractional microneedle RF (FMRF) treatments you can see a reduction in fat deposits, which can be explained by both thermal and simultaneous mechanical disruption of adipose cell membranes due to repeated mechanical trauma of a series of 3 microneedle RF treatments (**Fig. 3**).

KINNEY

The burn literature extends back to the late nineteenth century and has a few well-defined classic concepts. In the center of a burn wound with the greatest exposure to heat, there is a zone of necrosis. Outside of this circle, there is an annulus known as the zone of coagulation. Outside this is another annulus known as the zone of inflammation. Finally, there is another zone known as the normal zone. This zone represents tissue unheated or uninjured.

The Food and Drug Administration (FDA) has cleared essentially all RF devices under the category of soft tissue coagulation. There is no category for soft tissue inflammation. Most devices do not control the temperature and instead emit a blast of energy that may be controlled by time, fractional delivery to the tissues, focusing, microscopic needling, or similar methods. For these devices that cause coagulative necrosis, there is a dependence on the body's incredible resiliency and flexibility in healing capacity: the tissue injury–wound healing relationship.

For all energy-based devices there are the 4 classic zones of tissue in the treated tissue. It is just a matter of how far away from the hottest spot various cells are located, whether there

is a time-based, fractional, focused beam, needling-based or other treatment. Various cells fall into one of the 4 categories. Cells in the zone of coagulation undergo necrosis. Cells in the zone of inflammation likely undergo pyroptosis with or without apoptosis. FMRF possesses the capability to create mechanical poration of adipose cells in addition to electroporation of cell membranes.

Controlling the temperature by a thermistor and computer algorithm provides an alternative method for addressing tissue treatment with the added benefit of tissue selectivity. Under optimal conditions, because of temperature control, there is no zone of necrosis. Creating a zone of coagulation could be accomplished, if desired, by setting the temperature high enough, likely up to 100°C. Thus, the zone of inflammation can be larger without inner zones of necrosis and coagulation. In the zone of inflammation, pyroptosis would occur by design and could be controlled in intensity (**Fig. 4**).

SADICK

Research has shown that heating the dermis causes collagen coagulation resulting in immediate skin shrinkage and kick-starts the wound-healing process, a microinflammatory stimulation of fibroblasts, which produces new collagen, new elastin, and other substances, to enhance dermal structure. As new collagen replaces the old due to neocollagenesis and neoelastinogenesis, skin tightening occurs. Collagen denaturation occurs by heating the

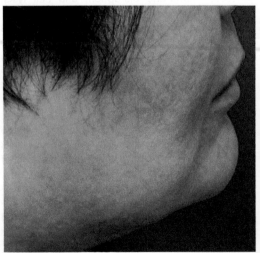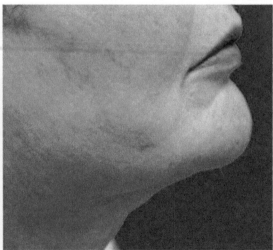

Fig. 3. Contour improvements in patient treated with FMRF shows reduction of adipose tissue, which may be due to both biochemical and mechanical poration of adipocyte cell membranes. Jowl fat evident preoperatively on left. Contour improvement postoperatively on right.

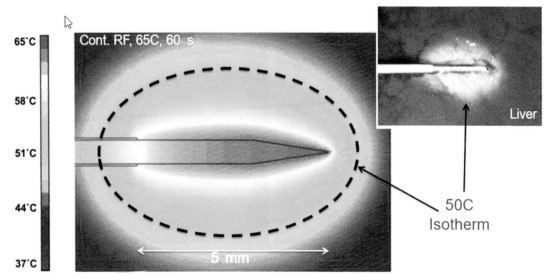

Fig. 4. Isotherm volume with pulsed RF at 20 W. CRFL, continuous radio frequency. (*Adapted from* Cosman ER Jr, Cosman ER Sr. Electric and thermal field effects in tissue around radiofrequency electrodes. Pain Med 2005;6(6):405–24; with permission.)

dermis to 40°C to 48°C, and collagen coagulation occurs around 55°C to 70°C. As the collagen coagulates and dehydrates, there is immediate tissue shrinkage. During the cooling stage of the treatment, as cellular membranes and tissue architecture have changed, a mild wound-healing response occurs. Necrosis is not expected as long as the temperatures do not remain too high for a prolonged time, but naturally there will be a few cells that undergo programmed cell death (apoptosis) and necrosis. The contribution of these processes to the effects of RF, however, are not severe or else treatments would result in visible scarring and ulcers due to an inflammatory reaction.[11] The term *pyroptosis*, although not widespread, may be an appropriate alternative to describing the RF mechanism of action, as it lies somewhat between apoptosis where cell death occurs and necrosis where cell death and profound inflammatory response is induced. In the case of fractional microneedling, there is controlled mechanical damage from the needling effect; but this has only beneficial consequences and synergistically enhances neocollagenesis and elastogenesis.[12] Penetration of the dermis with the microneedles has been demonstrated to mechanically stimulate fibroblasts to produce collagen, and this treatment exists as a standalone aesthetic modality without being paired to RF.

Question 3: Monopolar, bipolar, multipolar, multi-generator radiofrequency for the face and neck: how do you select the best radiofrequency device type to ensure the best clinical outcome?

GENTILE

In my practice, I have used various RF devices that cover most of the device designs that are available and are mentioned earlier. I think when considering the devices that will be selected for individual practices, the technology design and its overall effectiveness and patient satisfaction must be considered. In addition to polarity and generator design, the availability of temperature-monitoring thermistors and suction-assisted designs and contact cooling should be considered when evaluating these units for office use. I currently maintain 2 monopolar units, one with temperature control and one without. My main technology is a multipolar unit, and this large console unit is equipped with suction-assisted applicators for the face and body and is temperature controlled. I have 2 FMRF devices, one that is temperature controlled and one that is not temperature controlled. I also use a subcutaneous catheter-based temperature-controlled RF device, which is used for both skin tightening as well as contouring via thermal fat ablation.

My usual protocol when treating the face and neck involves using a temperature-controlled multipolar unit (**Fig. 5**) without suction, and I recommend a treatment protocol of at least 5 treatments. I find the suction unit to not be popular with patients and may occasionally leave them with low-grade bruising, which should not accompany noninvasive treatments. I would add that the medium-sized applicator is not ideal for treatment in the periocular

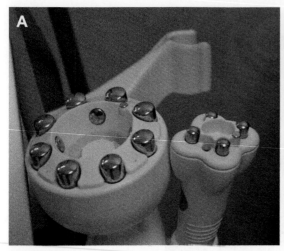
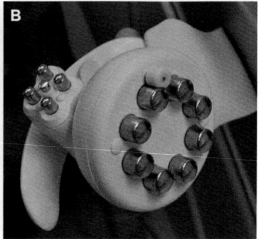

Fig. 5. Temperature-controlled unit demonstrating suction (*A*) and nonsuction (*B*) facial and body applicators/transducers.

region, and for this I would select the temperature-controlled small footprint applicator (**Fig. 6**) because of the superior mobility of the device in the periocular region. When treating the face and neck, it is important to consider what the RF treatment is to accomplish. Is it to improve the texture, to contour, or to tighten the skin? The level of invasiveness needs to be addressed. Although FMRF can accomplish more in terms of skin tightening and facial contouring, it requires local anesthetic and it may not be suitable for patients who want a noninvasive treatment.

KINNEY

There is overlap in the capability of various RF devices; however, the differences are sufficient to develop general approaches to treatment in the face. The mechanism can be divided into a few broad categories: (1) topical monopolar, nontemperature controlled; (2) topical monopolar, temperature controlled; (3) topical fractional without cooling; (4) topical fractional without cooling; (5) subcutaneous without temperature control; and (6) subcutaneous with temperature control.

Choosing a device for the face and neck depends on the severity of the condition, the skin

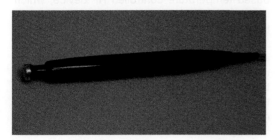

Fig. 6. Temperature-controlled small footprint applicator for periocular treatment.

thickness, Fitzpatrick skin type/pigmentation, and the anatomic area, among other factors.[13]

For smoothing, tightening, and progressive collagen stimulation in younger patients without advanced solar and aging-related degeneration, repeated treatments with topical handpieces at lower settings are adequate. A pure monopolar RF device, such as Pellevé (Cynosure, Westford, MA), can improve the face incrementally over time. Usually, 3 to 5 treatments are required at 2- to 3-week intervals. Temperature achieved on the skin depends on the rhythm and speed of the handpiece movement. Exilis (BTL Industries, Prague, Czech Republic) adds ultrasound to the RF for an intended improved result. ThermiSmooth (ThermiAesthetics/Almirall, Barcelona, Spain) is a temperature-controlled device that improves the consistency of energy delivery because of the computer generator algorithm that senses the skin at 2 Hz during the treatment.

In the quest for enhanced results, higher energy can be delivered with higher temperatures. However, this leaves the challenge of pain control and prevention of excessive burn. The fractional, microneedle, and focused methods cause burns by design, as mentioned earlier. Thermage (Solta, Hayward, CA) is indicated in patients with moderate/severe laxity and rhytids in the forehead, cheeks, midface, jaw line, neck, and under the eyes. In the early days of this device, patients were treated under intravenous sedation or general anesthesia for pain control; however, this leads to an unacceptable incidence of burns. Later iterations switched to treating awake patients. A simultaneous pulse of fractionated RF was delivered along with a small jet of cryogen to prevent injury to the skin. This method allows for more intensive energy delivery and more demonstrable results in advanced skin laxity and rhytids. Other fractional devices create spaced vertical columns of thermal necrosis and coagulation. Neal has mentioned 2.

In my practice, I tend to use ThermiTight (ThermiAesthetics) because of its selectively in targeting tissues without causing necrosis. The advantages are the minimal cost for disposable tips; the ability to treat deep to the nerves, fascia, fibro-septal network, and subcutaneous fat; as well as the ability to tighten the dermis and epidermis. Disadvantages include a demanding learning curve, the requirement for knowing the internal anatomy in detail, and an increased risk of nerve injury when not planned as part of the procedure. If desired, nerves can be targeted and neurotoxins would not be required. The duration of a nerve lesion can extend from 9 to 12 months with 2 to 3 lesions per nerve up to a permanent result with 8 to 10 lesions and a 1.5- to 2.0-cm gap in the nerve.

SADICK

Currently, there is a surplus of RF devices for face and neck rejuvenation; selecting the right ones for your practice can be daunting for both novice and seasoned clinicians. Technologies differ not only in the number of electrodes and mode of RF-energy delivery but also in their capacity to be paired with other energy sources, such as ultrasound, light, pulsed-electromagnetic fields, and so forth. The reality is that newer devices will continue to enter the market that will allow us to treat our patients even more safely and with greater efficacy than the devices currently available; but regardless, there are overarching best practices that can guide appropriate device selection. Any clinical practice should have more than one RF device for skin rejuvenation to cater to different skin types and dermatologic indications. A pure monopolar RF device, such as Pellevé or Thermage, is necessary for treating skin that presents moderate/severe laxity and rhytids in the forehead, cheeks, midface, jaw line, neck, and under the eyes.[14] The volumetric heating action rendered by these devices stimulates denaturation/recoiling of collagen fibers and stimulates extracellular matrix production that improves skin elasticity. Bipolar, multipolar, and multi-generator devices do not deliver RF energy to the deep dermis and, thus, are more appropriate for younger patients looking to prevent the signs of aging, for patients with mild laxity, or for off-face indications. Another device necessary for a clinical practice is a fractional RF device, such as the Intensif RF (EndyMed, New York, NY) or the Venus Viva (Venus Concept,

Toronto, Canada). These devices are ideal for patients of any skin type presenting with dyschromias, large pores, scarring, and deep wrinkles. Fractional RF delivers energy through an array of microscopic columns of spatially confined thermal injury (microscopic thermal zones), allowing the untreated areas of tissue to serve as reservoirs fueling a more rapid dermal remodeling process. In my practice, I tend to use Thermage in patients with moderate laxity usually in conjunction with soft tissue fillers and neurotoxins. For patients with more complex and heterogeneous face/neck skin manifestations, I usually recommend a series of fractional Venus Viva treatments to even out the skin tone and texture and then assess the subsequent needs for volumization or additional treatments for laxity. Needless to say, a spot check is required before any treatment, as each patient's skin can react differently, even unexpectedly, to the proposed recommendation.

Question 4: Do you agree or disagree: using the same number of radiofrequency treatments and same type of radiofrequency device in the face and neck guarantees homogeneous skin tightening effects?

GENTILE

I would disagree with this statement, and it really relates to the highly variable results of RF in patients. There have been shortcomings with RF tightening devices, including inconsistent clinical outcomes; the question arises, why are there inconsistent results and variability among patient outcomes? Variability could be related to different devices, treatment protocols, body area treated, and patient selection. Patient age, degree of laxity, history of smoking, ethnicity, body mass index, and individual patient pain threshold could all possibly contribute to patients' response to tightening devices. It is well accepted that the energy that enters the treated target tissue relates directly to the tissue impedance at the time of treatment. It is also known that tissue and, more specifically, skin impedance varies between different individuals and in the same individuals between body sites and according to the real-time skin humidity. Considering the treatment protocol involving the same device treatments, data confirm the existence of large fluctuations in skin impedance between individual patients and during nonablative treatment sessions in the same patient.

KINNEY

All heat is not alike. Perhaps we have not studied the physiologic response enough; however, the mechanism of RF is clearly different than laser. Subcutaneous temperature-controlled RF can improve the skin pores and fine laxity by applying RF immediately deep to the dermis with resultant heating and contraction superficially. The temperature-controlled approach, especially, has the advantage of acceptability in Fitzpatrick skin types I to VI. Although safe in these patients, the contradistinction is RF does not have the ability to improve dyschromia. Ablative lasers have a high risk of pigmentary damage. It is just not feasible to treat all skin types with ablative lasers; moreover, nonablative lasers are not able to achieve the degree of deep tissue tightening as RF or the cutaneous tissue tightening as ablative laser.

Although ablative lasers are superior for acne scars, lasers of any kind have essentially no impact on the fibro-septal network or fascia. Overtightening the skin to lift the neck or face creates an unnatural, unsatisfying appearance and may lead to permanently damaged, desiccated, atretic skin.

Question 5: What are the best ways to address tissue selectively in the face and neck with radiofrequency?

GENTILE

Conventional RF devices may have difficulties in targeting tissues selectively with traditional transcutaneous approaches. When I am suggesting selective targeting of tissues, I would be considering dermal collagen, adipocytes, and the fibrous septal network as targets for treatment. For many years, the tissue tightening component was thought to be primarily dermal collagen. More recent studies have indicated that soft tissue contraction at the level of the fibrous septal network in the interstitial space between the deep dermis and the subcutaneous fat layer may be the best location for energy deposition. With this area as a target, it is easy to understand why selectively treating at this depth would be a problem with conventional devices. To reach therapeutic levels in the deep dermis, near burn level temperatures would need to be maintained at the cutaneous level. One option for reducing superficial cutaneous treatment temperatures would be to use contact cooling. In some instances, continuous contact cooling permits the RF energy to pass by the skin without injuring it and to then accumulate, in the deeper dermis, adipocytes and peri-adipocyte collagen. One interesting physical phenomenon is that on the surface of the skin heat evaporates because of ambient conditions. In the interstitial space, evaporation or dissipation of the deep thermal energy does not

occur and may in some cases permit the deep temperatures to exceed the superficial temperatures. Conventional thinking does not always permit us to think that the deep temperature can be greater than the superficial or skin temperature, but contact cooling may accommodate this as well as the lack of heat dissipation in the closed interstitial space.

When considering the obstructionist characteristics of the epidermis in permitting energies that can accomplish skin tightening, collagen structural change and remodeling, and adipocyte alterations with contour changes, the best current option is to bypass the epidermis with either catheter-based RF energy or with FMRF. Both catheter-based RF and microneedle devices are able to bypass the epidermis to deliver the structurally altering energies to the fibrous septal network and the adipocyte level of the interstitial space.

KINNEY

Tissue selectivity cannot be easily addressed by cutaneous devices. They primarily treat the epidermis and dermis. Heating in deeper layers is minimally therapeutic and more limited. To compensate for this, multiple treatments over time are chosen but do not adequately address deeper layers. Tissue selectivity is addressed best by temperature control but only when the energy is delivered subcutaneously directly into the desired layer. This technique demands an intricate knowledge of the anatomy and is more challenging without surgical expertise. The differing tolerance of tissues to temperature and the targeting of layers based on this temperature is a new enhancement in our treatment armamentarium.

The topical devices achieve results but generally require multiple treatments over several months. Unfortunately, even spacing the treatments over time does not provide much tissue selectivity. Combining modalities, like RF and ultrasound, has shown some benefit. This combination may be performed with 2 different devices or with a single device like Exilis. To achieve tissue recontouring, injection of fillers and toxins can be added to the energy-based devices.

The ThermiTight probe has been successfully used as a one-time treatment of the dermis and epidermis from underneath, the fibro-septal network a few millimeters deep, and the supraplatysmal fat deeper. In addition, muscles like the orbicularis, frontalis, procerus, and nasalis can be treated directly to shorten and contract them or by ThermiRase to relax and smooth them like a toxin. More interestingly, ThermiTight and

ThermiRase can be performed at the same time to shorten, smooth, AND relax the muscle. This procedure is most commonly achieved in platysma bands but has been done in the frontalis, orbicularis oculi, procerus, nasalis, and mentalis. Stimulating collagen production seems to be an accompanying effect of all these treatments.

SADICK

The anatomy and pathophysiology of aging is different in the face and neck, and treatment protocols are subsequently quite distinct. Patients requesting face and neck rejuvenation often present a diverse gamut of dermatologic signs that require different treatment modalities. The neck, as opposed to the face, does not have thick adipose compartments to cushion the bones, and thus the skin loses its elasticity that manifests as sagging earlier than that seen in the face. Moreover, the neck is often neglected in daily skincare routine, and is overly exposed to external and internal aging stimuli. Neck rejuvenation for cases of mild/moderate severity usually requires 2 to 3 treatments in monthly intervals with a pure RF device, such as Thermage or Pellevé, as improvement of laxity is the main goal of treatment. Patients with severe neck sagging who do not wish to undergo surgical neck lift can benefit from the newest generation of minimally invasive RF technologies, such as ThermiTight. ThermiTight uses a tiny probe to go under the skin and delivers RF energy directly to the dermal layer, stimulating collagen production. Only one treatment is usually needed, which requires local anesthesia; but results so far are long-standing and progressive. In the face, depending on the individual, treatments may involve a series of fractional RF sessions for patients with textural issues (enlarged pores, deep rhytids, acne scars) or a monopolar RF for mild/moderate laxity combined with fillers/toxins. Another combination I find successful in terms of efficacy and patients' satisfaction is to do RF to the face and ultrasound (Ulthera, Merz, Frankfurt, Germany) to the neck and chest in one session.[15]

Question 6: What temperatures are indicated for nerve ablation, tissue tightening, skin rejuvenation, and stimulating an inflammatory response?

GENTILE

Both in vitro and in vivo studies have demonstrated that heat stress can directly induce cell death and tissue injury. The mechanisms of direct thermal injury of cells and tissue ablation includes carbonization, water vaporization, thermal denaturation of proteins, and cell membrane rupture. Some tissue components denature or dissociate at lower temperatures and are considered heat sensitive, whereas others denature at higher temperatures and are considered heat resistant. In relative terms of heat sensitivity, fat is more sensitive than collagen, which is more sensitive than neural tissue. Nerve ablation via thermal RF ablation (RFA) is generally carried out at 80°C for 90 seconds. However, one study suggests nerve ablation at 90°C was more effective; hence, a range of 80°C to 90°C is used. For superficial skin rejuvenation, the use of temperature-controlled devices at 43°C to 44°C maintained for 10 minutes has been associated with skin rejuvenation effects due to the dermal collagen thermal effects. For skin tightening that is a continuation of soft tissue contraction, treatment of the dermis and fibrous septal network should fall in the range of 55°C to 68°C. Some studies have suggested that 67°C for 3 seconds is ideal. With regard to inflammation following thermal injury, it has been reported that exposure to temperatures greater than 49°C to 50°C compromises cellular structures and function, leading to rapid necrotic cell death in less than 5 minutes. This temperature range is the dividing line for apoptosis (noninflammatory) cell death and necrosis (inflammatory cell death). The release of intracellular content after cellular membrane damage is the cause of inflammation in necrosis. There are many causes of necrosis, including injury, infection, cancer, infarction, toxins, and inflammation. It is clear that when cells die they set in motion several important processes. One is the rapid recruitment of innate immune components from the blood as part of a process we recognize as inflammation. Another parallel process is the mobilization of highly specific T- and B-cell defenses from more distal sites.

KINNEY

The largest portion of the literature reflects experience with energy-based devices and mentions joules per square centimeter instead of temperature. This demands continual evaluation of tissue response after each pass of the treatment. However, there is an inherent limitation of calibrating the tissue response by this approach.

A panel of 11 expert physicians convened a consensus conference in October 2016 in Southlake, Texas with doctors from plastic and facial plastic surgery, dermatology, and other aesthetic physicians. Before the meeting, a comprehensive review of the literature was performed. Literature revealed 10 different technologies for neck rejuvenation, and more than 1000 individuals were queried for treatment algorithms used in their clinics. These results have been submitted for publication as of this writing, and the emphasis was on temperature control for greater tissue selectivity.

Ferguson[16] found about 23% symmetric cross-sectional area reduction of the skin ($P<.001$) in abdominoplasty specimens treated with subcutaneous temperature-controlled RF to a target of 51°C. Four lines were created in each of 48 samples. An additional 4 lines resulted in about 3% additional contraction. The pass was performed at the level of the Scarpa fascia.[16]

Key[17] treated 35 patients in a 3-cm^2 area of the neck every 2 minutes at 50°C to 60°C while maintaining the skin at 42°C. He found a postprocedure improvement of 0.78 on a 4-point laxity scale ($P<.001$) at 3 months.

In a 1064/130-nm laser, DiBernardo and colleagues[18] found epidermal and dermal injury at skin temperatures of 47°C concomitant with 50°C to 55°C temperatures at a 5-mm depth. This temperature stimulates an inflammatory response. Blistering occurred at more than 58°C.

Nerve ablation lasted longer than 12 months in 78% of 27 patients as reported in an article by Kim and colleagues.[19] My personal experience with approximately 75 patients shows heating to 85°C with a 22-g, 5-cm exposed tip probe for 1 minute and creating about 5 lesions over a distance of 2 cm provides more than 1 year of results and in some cases multiple years.

In my experience with more than 600 cases, 85°C is indicated for nerves, 70°C for treating subcutaneous fat, 60°C for connective tissue, and about 43°C to 48°C for connective stimulation with neocollagenesis.

SADICK

Therapeutic temperatures for RF delivery for safe outcomes in indications such as skin rejuvenation/tightening is shown to be in the 55°C to 68°C range to generate an appropriate response. When treating patients with RF devices for aesthetic improvements, safe temperatures must be maintained in the epidermis at less than the 40°C mark or else epidermal damage is caused, which negatively affects wound healing and could result in postinflammatory hyperpigmentation. Moreover, prolonged high temperatures (more than 68°C) can cause tissue necrosis and lead to inflammatory-mediated injury due to the triggering of a strong wound healing/immune response. For nerve ablation, RFA is a well-established treatment modality and a wide range (70°C–90°C) has been used. Although there is a paucity of research evaluating the optimal

temperature for this treatment, one study showed significant functional improvement associated with a temperature of 90°C compared with 80°C, with no added risk of complications.

Question 7: How have you changed your use of energy-based technologies over the last 5 years?

GENTILE

My evolution in RF technologies was essentially a wider embrace of all the technologies, as the device engineering and results improved over the past 5 years. One of the interesting things about all technology devices is that when they are released, the dosimetry is not always optimal for patient results. The reason for this is that many FDA studies are performed with the objective to show effectiveness (not necessarily the best results) but primarily to limit complications so that the device will be approved. When the devices are released, the settings used are the ones used in the studies. Ultimately, it is then up to the aesthetic community to determine how to get the optimal results with the devices. This determination can be hashed out in publications, meeting communications, or user groups. About 10 years ago, I introduced subcutaneous laser surgery of the face and neck with SmartLipo (Cynosure, Waltham, MA); it was in conjunction with this and the work of other plastic surgeons and dermatologists that the actual thermodynamics of interactions of energy-based devices and tissue became more apparent. Thus, the genre of thermoplastic treatment grew to include interstitial (subcutaneous) devices and microneedle delivery devices all having RF options. The single most important development over the past few years is that thermosensors have been integrated in the delivery tips and capacitors. In some of these devices, the engineering is an amazing technological feat. In the Profound device (Syneron-Candela, Yokneam Israel), sensors are integrated on a 32-gauge needle and provide real-time thermal monitoring of the subcutaneous or dermal temperatures present as the device operates depending on what handpiece is attached. So I have embraced more devices as the technology improved the delivery approach (interstitial or transepidermal needle) and also the temperature sensors' deployment so that the end points of treatment can be better appreciated. My current devices include the ones mentioned by other investigators, including ThermiTight and ThermiSmooth, Profound, Infini (Lutronic, Burlington, MA), Aluma (Lumenis, Israel), and Venus Viva and Venus Legacy.

SADICK

Five years ago, my main go-to RF device was a first-generation unipolar device; I used it mainly for facial laxity. Over the years, I became an early adopter of the new-generation devices, for example, the multi-generator RF (EndyMed 3DEEP), the multipolar RF combined with pulsed electromagnetic fields (Venus Legacy), the nano-fractional RF (Venus Viva), and recently the temperature-controlled RF (ThermiRF, ThermiAesthetics, Irving, TX).[20–22] The overarching theme with every year that passed is my increased use of the new-generation devices for a plethora of face and off-face indications and the gradual displacement of lasers in their favor. For example, instead of a fractional laser for acne scars, I now prefer to use a microneedling RF device. Or instead of multiple passes and treatments with a monopolar RF for treating cellulite/laxity, I now perform a single treatment with a temperature-controlled RF device. The new technologies have reduced the treatment time, cause less pain compared with the first-generation devices, have no downtime, and have superior efficacy.

KINNEY

The first wave of aesthetic laser and RF devices that became widespread starting about 15 to 20 years ago was transcutaneous devices at lower power. The initial experience was encouraging; however, not only were energy levels not well worked out but also the results were variable. Patient selection was viewed as key, but the actual process of selecting patients was not understood. Most patients had excellent results and some little. Millions of patients were treated effectively. However, in order to increase response rates, energy was increased; but this came with increased risk of burns and other problems. In the early 2000s began the era of subcutaneous devices, first with laser as noted by Richard and subsequently with RF and other techniques. Transcutaneous devices still remain an essential and popular part of the clinical armamentarium. The concept of temperature control was well known for decades. However, the first widespread use in medicine in my view was by radiologists and pain management experts for treatment in the spine for chronic pain syndromes, an area where broad energy delivery via joules per square centimeter was truly dangerous with a risk of devastating motor nerve injury. More than a half million treatments took place starting about 10 years ago. Using the ThermiTight (ThermiRF)[20–22] procedure and then other similar techniques, my clinic popularized everyday use of tissue selectivity and temperature control for aesthetic enhancement, first in the face and subsequently throughout the body. The challenge of patient selection has not been solved completely, but results have been improved. Several excellent devices are available, and many have added temperature control in the last few years, including FaceTite and BodyTite (InMode, Israel) in addition to those excellent devices mentioned by Richard and Neal. Although temperature control has been a major advance, it requires improvement and supplementation. How do we know when we have treated enough, when we are done? The major treatment paradigm is of tissue injury/healing response for rejuvenation. Our medical literature abounds with articles from one field or the other. However, the challenge of pairing the two in a predictive and reliable way is currently overwhelming. How do we predict how long the tissue will take after treatment to be optimal? How much should we injure the tissue? Which tissues should we injure and which not? How should we be more selective? The questions are myriad. The future compels us to develop and introduce new methods of tissue monitoring and selectively, beyond temperature. This development may mean the use of real-time biochemical sensors like pH, inflammatory markers, real-time contractility gauges, and others.

REFERENCES

1. Goldberg DJ. Nonablative laser technology radiofrequency. Aesthet Surg J 2004;24(2):180–1.
2. Koch RJ. Radiofrequency nonablative tissue tightening. Facial Plast Surg Clin North Am 2004;12(3): 339–46, vi.
3. Ruiz-Esparza J, Gomez JB. The medical face lift: a noninvasive, nonsurgical approach to tissue tightening in facial skin using nonablative radiofrequency. Dermatol Surg 2003;29(4):325–32 [discussion: 332].
4. Kushikata N, Negishi K, Tezuka Y, et al. Non-ablative skin tightening with radiofrequency in Asian skin. Lasers Surg Med 2005;36(2):92–7.
5. Sadick N, Sorhaindo L. The radiofrequency frontier: a review of radiofrequency and combined radiofrequency pulsed-light technology in aesthetic medicine. Facial Plast Surg 2005;21(2):131–8.
6. Sadick NS, Sato M, Palmisano D, et al. In vivo animal histology and clinical evaluation of multisource fractional radiofrequency skin resurfacing (FSR) applicator. J Cosmet Laser Ther 2011; 13(5):204–9.
7. Sadick NS, Trelles MA. A clinical, histological, and computer-based assessment of the Polaris LV, combination diode, and radiofrequency system,

for leg vein treatment. Lasers Surg Med 2005; 36(2):98–104.

8. Gonzalez-Suarez A, Gutierrez-Herrera E, Berjano E, et al. Thermal and elastic response of subcutaneous tissue with different fibrous septa architectures to RF heating: numerical study. Lasers Surg Med 2015; 47(2):183–95.

9. Fink SL, Cookson BT. Apoptosis, pyroptosis, and necrosis: mechanistic description of dead and dying eukaryotic cells. Infect Immun 2005;73(4):1907–16.

10. Kepp O, Galluzzi L, Zitvogel L, et al. Pyroptosis - a cell death modality of its kind? Eur J Immunol 2010;40(3):627–30.

11. Fritz K, Salavastru C. Ways of noninvasive facial skin tightening and fat reduction. Facial Plast Surg 2016; 32(3):276–82.

12. Sadick N, Rothaus KO. Minimally invasive radiofrequency devices. Clin Plast Surg 2016;43(3):567–75.

13. Jones IT, Guiha I, Goldman MP, et al. A randomized evaluator-blinded trial comparing subsurface monopolar radiofrequency with microfocused ultrasound for lifting and tightening of the neck. Dermatol Surg 2017. [Epub ahead of print].

14. Fabi SG, Niwa Massaki AB, Goldman MP. Clinical efficacy and safety of a monopolar radiofrequency device with comfort pulse technology for the treatment of facial and neck laxity in men. Skinmed 2016;14(3): 181–5.

15. DiBernardo BE, DiBernardo G, Pozner JN. Subsurface laser and radiofrequency for face and body rejuvenation. Clin Plast Surg 2016;43(3):527–33.

16. Ferguson J. Effects of subdermal monopolar RF energy on abdominoplasty flaps. J Drugs Dermatol 2016;15(1):55–8.

17. Key DJ. Integration of thermal imaging with subsurface radiofrequency thermistor heating for the purpose of skin tightening and contour improvement: a retrospective review of clinical efficacy. J Drugs Dermatol 2014;13(12):1485–9.

18. DiBernardo BE, Reyes J, Chen B. Evaluation of tissue thermal effects from 1064/1320-nm laser-assisted lipolysis and its clinical implications. J Cosmet Laser Ther 2009;11(2):62–9.

19. Kim JH, Jeong JW, Son D, et al. Percutaneous selective radiofrequency nerve ablation for glabellar frown lines. Aesthet Surg J 2011;31(7):747–55.

20. Krueger N, Levy H, Sadick NS. Safety and efficacy of a new device combining radiofrequency and low-frequency pulsed electromagnetic fields for the treatment of facial rhytides. J Drugs Dermatol 2012;11(11):1306–9.

21. Krueger N, Sadick NS. New-generation radiofrequency technology. Cutis 2013;91(1):39–46.

22. Sadick N. Bipolar radiofrequency for facial rejuvenation. Facial Plast Surg Clin North Am 2007;15(2): 161–7, v.

The Superficial Musculoaponeurotic System and Other Considerations in Rejuvenation of the Lower Face and Neck

William H. Truswell IV, MD[a,b,c],*, Harrison C. Putman III, MD[d], Stephen W. Perkins, MD[e,f], Nathan Johnson, MD[g]

KEYWORDS

- SMAS • Platysmaplasty • The heavy face • Imbrication • Facelift

KEY POINTS

- Visible anterior platysma banding can be addressed by various techniques and midline platysma plication or imbrication.
- Patients presenting with anatomic variations such as heavy face and neck or midface volume deficiency may require detailed counseling and realistic expectations, as well as condition-specific operative maneuvers for optimum results.
- Patient satisfaction is perhaps the single most important metric in a successful aesthetic facial plastic surgical practice.
- Proper vectoring techniques are critical to successful facelift outcomes and longevity.

Question 1: What is your go-to technique for handling anterior platysma banding when performing a lower face and neck lift?

TRUSWELL

That there are many approaches to managing anterior platysma bands attests to the frustrations facial plastic surgeons have with the early recurrence of the banding.[1–4] Nascent face lift surgeons have the lessons of their residencies and fellowships in the forefront of their minds. With time and growing experience, the issue of this problem will become apparent. Meetings, seminars, courses, and videos will show the plethora of procedures addressing this problem. Eventually, a personal solution will be found and it is hoped that outcomes will improve.

This author's go-to techniques is the corset platysmaplasty. The patient is marked in the sitting position. The estimated area of submental undermining, the top of the thyroid cartilage, the

Disclosure: The authors have nothing to disclose.
[a] Private Practice, I23 Union Street, Suite 100, Easthampton, MA 01027, USA; [b] Private Practice, 2114 Landfall Way, Johns Island, Charleston, SC 29455, USA; [c] Facial Plastic Surgery, Division of Otolaryngology, Department of Surgery, University of Connecticut School of Medicine, Farmington, CT, USA; [d] Department of Otolaryngology, SIU Medical School, Springfield, IL, USA; [e] Private Practise, Indianapolis, IN, USA; [f] Private Practise, Meridian Plastic Surgery Center, Meridian Plastic Surgeons, 170 West 106th Street, Indianapolis, IN 46290, USA; [g] Private Practice, Facial Plastic and Reconstructive Surgery, Ear, Nose and Throat Specialty Care, Minneapolis, MN 55404, USA
* Corresponding author. I23 Union Street, Suite 100, Easthampton, MA 01027.
E-mail address: bill.truswell@gmail.com

Panel discussion

1. What is your go-to technique for handling anterior platysma banding when performing a lower face and neck lift?

2. A moderately overweight patient desires a lower face and neck lift. The patient has no intention of losing weight. Will you offer this patient surgery and why or why not? What is your approach to the heavy face and neck and how do you counsel this patient?

3. What is your mainstay procedure for repositioning the superficial musculoaponeurotic system and how, if at all, would you vary your approach?

4. A patient with moderate jowl and wattle formation desires a facelift. This patient also has marked sunken cheeks. What is your recommendation for rejuvenation of the lower face and neck in this patient? If you recommend an ancillary procedure and the patient refuses and only wants the facelift, would you proceed? If so, why? If not, why not?

5. What do you consider a successful outcome in facial rejuvenation? From "Hello" to "Goodbye", and technique aside, what is your philosophy on communicating with and educating your patients that contributes to a successful outcome?

6. How has your approach to rejuvenation of the lower face and neck changed over the last 5 years?

cervicomental angle, and the submental crease are delineated (**Fig. 1**). With the patient recumbent in the operating room, monitored anesthesia is commenced. The incision line is infiltrated with 1% lidocaine with 1:100,000 epinephrine and the area of the anterior flap elevation is infiltrated with 0.5% lidocaine and 1:100,000 epinephrine.

After 10 minutes have elapsed, a 2-cm to 3-cm incision is made just beneath the submental crease. The anterior neck skin is elevated by blunt scissor dissection with care being taken to leave a thin layer of fat on the flap if possible (**Fig. 2**). A pearl to keep in mind is that the tips of the scissors should always be seen beneath the flaps during this blind dissection, which provides assurance that the surgeon is safely in the correct plane (**Fig. 3**). Open liposuction is performed as needed in the submental area and beneath the body of the mandible.

Following liposuction, I elevate each platysma band for 3 to 4 cm from the mentum to the top of the thyroid cartilage. If one or both platysma bands is heavily redundant, I resect the medial edge as needed, usually up to 1 cm. I then divide the elevated bands laterally for 2 to 3 cm at the cervicomental junction (**Fig. 4**). I suture the bands together above this cut with 2-0 polydioxanone (PDO) Quill barbed absorbable suture (Angiotech Pharmaceuticals, Vancouver, Canada). The suture is double armed with the barbs facing away from the needles. I use a continuous simple running stitch from the cervicomental junction to the mentum with both needles. The barbs anchor into the tissue and no knot is needed. The incision is closed with 4-0 polyglactin 910 subcuticularly

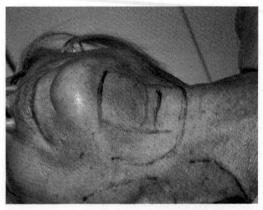

Fig. 1. Area of submental dissection. Incision in submental crease, hyoid bone, anterior platysma bands are marked.

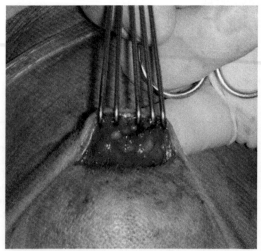

Fig. 2. Visible thin fat layer on the undersurface of the submental fat.

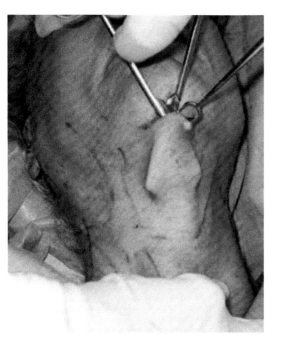

Fig. 3. Elevation of the submental flap. Keeping the scissor tips evident during elevation ensures dissection is in the safe subcutaneous plane.

and 6-0 fast-absorbing plain gut cutaneous sutures.

For treating the lateral cheeks and neck I perform a sub–superficial musculoaponeurotic system (sub-SMAS) procedure. The strong lift and imbrication of the SMAS creates the effect of tightening a corset on the anterior neck (**Fig. 5**).

PUTMAN

Over the lifespan of my career as a facial plastic surgeon, I have used a variety of techniques to address anterior platysma banding in different situations, including the classic techniques described by Feldman,[5] Guyuron and colleages,[6] and Henly and colleagues.[7] Currently I most often use the Kelly clamp technique described by my coauthor, Dr Stephen Perkins, and others.[7] However, I modify this as needed to perform subplatysmal midline fat sculpting before closure. I always create a freshly trimmed medial edge of platysma muscle on each side and use permanent sutures (3-0 or 4-0 Ethibond) with a doubly reinforced closure whenever possible, similar to the technique described by Feldman.[5] I do this in order to reinforce the midline repair and attempt to prevent recurrent banding in the future. I avoid excessive tension on this closure because I firmly believe this contributes to the eventual recurrence of banding. I also perform a horizontal back cut for 2 to 3 cm at the level of the hyoid bone or mentocervical break. I do not advocate complete platysma transection because I believe this contributes to postsurgical deformities including so-called widow shading, and so forth.

PERKINS

One of the first things surgeons should do in the preoperative evaluation for treating the neck in facelifting is to understand that the primary concern of most patients is improvement of necklines that have begun to show significant signs of aging, and this bothers them even more than relaxation of the cheek and jawline. The other part to understand in causes of aging of the neck is that the loss of elasticity in the skin is commensurate and in conjunction with the loss of elasticity and sagging of the platysma muscle. The skin and platysma muscle lose their elasticity, and the effect of gravity creates skin and platysmal banding, even if it is hidden with hereditary and dietary lipoptosis. It is my opinion, and my experience, that surgeons

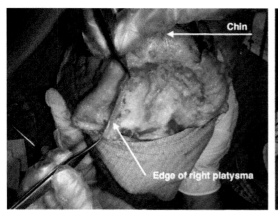
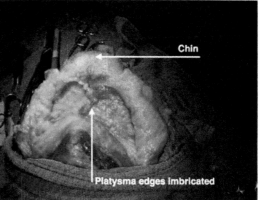

Fig. 4. Cadaver dissection. (*Left*) Edge of right platysma dissected. (*Right*)

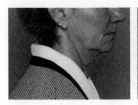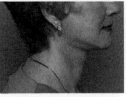

Fig. 5. Before (*left*) and after (*right*) views of an ideal 60-year-old patient with a very good surgical result.

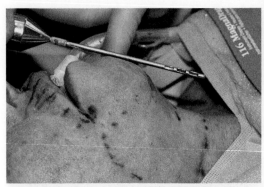

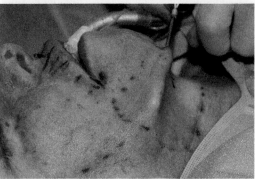

Fig. 6. A 3-mm round liposuction cannula with 3 rectangular holes on one side is used to preelevate tunnels in a radial fashion into the jowl, submandibular, and submental region in a fanlike fashion from the left side all the way to the right side.

must pay attention to treating the laxity of the platysma muscle to achieve a long-lasting result in the neck that is satisfying to the patient and minimizes the need for any tuck-up procedures by the surgeon. This outcome requires, in most cases, full elevation of the skin and separating it from the platysma muscle. Before skin elevation, any lipoptosis of the submental, submandibular, and even jowl areas should be removed with careful and judicious liposuction techniques. Rarely do I use direct excision of fatty tissue. It is important to leave a layer of adipose tissue on the undermined skin, because it creates a smoother contour in the neck and jawline and prevents the potential for dermal banding of the skin.

In my opinion and experience of more than 34 years of performing facelift procedures, the foundation of the facelift procedure requires treatment of the neck first. This requirement means that, before posterior suspension of the platysma muscle, I create a firm end-to-end platysmal imbrication of the anterior borders of the shortened platysma muscle. This imbrication creates a full-neck sling that can then be posteriorly suspended, creating a sharp, tight neckline that will last at least 10 to 15 years and may never recur to the preoperative condition.[8]

The procedure is started by making a 3-cm to 4-cm incision in the submental crease, followed by a short elevation of the skin to expose the subcutaneous tissue. A small 3-mm round liposuction cannula with 3 rectangular holes on one side is used to preelevate tunnels into jowl in a radial fashion into the jowl, submandibular, and submental region in a fanlike fashion from the left side all the way to the right side (**Fig. 6**). Once pretunneling has been accomplished, judicious application of liposuction at 1 atmospheric pressure is performed. Care is taken not to overliposuction the jowl but to moderately aggressively liposuction the submandibular fat pocket. Surgeons do not want to create dimpling in the jowl or dermal banding in the anterior neck. Symmetric and adequate liposuction is accomplished using the nondominant hand to palpate the fatty tissues underneath the surface of the skin, lifting the tissues and excess fat, feeding it into the cannula. The cannula

is rotated 180°, left to right, during these in-and-out maneuvers. Surgeons also want to avoid excessive liposuction to prevent the exposure of ptotic submandibular glands. Ptotic submandibular glands occasionally occur and may be visible after proper neck surgery, despite tightening of the platysmal muscle as a corset sling. I do not believe excising submandibular glands is an appropriate part of a cosmetic neck/facelift.

I favor the use of a 14-cm (5.5-inch) Kelly clamp technique for the submental platysmaplasty. It is performed under direct vision through the incision just anterior to the submental natural crease. The skin of the neck is undermined with Kahn beveled facelift dissection scissors in an advanced spreading technique and then the cutting of small bridges of remaining tissue. This dissection is more easily performed after having passed the liposuction cannula first. The elevation of the skin is continued past the cervicomental angle to the thyroid cartilage and all the way laterally to the anterior border of the sternocleidomastoid bilaterally. The looseness of the anterior platysma and any remaining adipose tissues is easily visualized and picked up with Griffiths-Brown forceps. These forceps pick up the anterior platysma bands, as well as any excess subplatysmal fat that is redundant in the midline. A large curved Kelly clamp is then used to tighten these tissues in the anterior midline (**Fig. 7**). I clamp this tissue 2 to 3 times to ensure that I am tightening as much as the soft tissue looseness allows me. Then I am assured I can easily immediately suture the anterior borders back together in an imbricating fashion. No further dissection underneath the platysma muscle is required, and this also prevents any kind of so-called cobra deformity by resection of too much subplatysmal fat. The excision of the tissue starts at the level of the submental incision and moves directly to the cervicomental angle. It is a sequential cauterization, excision, and immediate suturing with a mattressing buried 3-0 Vicryl suture (Ethicon, Somerville, NJ) (**Fig. 8**). This sequential excision suturing is done to the submental crease down to the cervicomental angle. Occasionally, the suturing is extended across the cervicomental angle for a smooth contour, similar to described by Feldman.[9] However, most of the time, to create a better cervicomental angle than the patient had preoperatively, a wedge excision of the anterior border of the platysma muscle is performed for as much as 1 to 3 cm at the cervicomental angle (**Fig. 9**). The combined anterior borders of the platysmal muscle with any subplatysmal fat are then excised completely. If there is fat at the cervicomental angle in the subplatysmal plane, it is directly contoured at that time. This occurrence is much less common.

In a patient who has a very heavy neck, such as a man, or in a patient with overly fatty tissues (**Fig. 10**), the 3-0 Vicryl sutures (Ethicon) are supported with 3-0 permanent braided suture, such as Mersilene (Ethicon). Earlier in my practice, I used permanent 2-0 Ethibond (Ethicon) sutures but suture extrusion did occur in 3% to 4% of

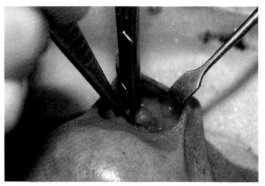
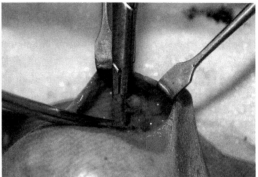
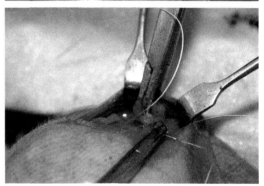

Fig. 8. The excess tissue is then sequentially cauterized and excised with immediate suturing using a buried 3-0 mattress Vicryl suture. (*Courtesy of* Ethicon, Inc, Somerville, NJ.)

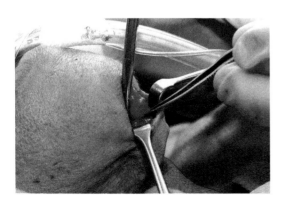

Fig. 7. A large curved Kelly clamp is then used to tighten these tissues in the anterior midline.

my patients. To this date, over the last 15 years, no Mersilene (Ethicon) sutures have extruded.

At this juncture of the facelift procedure, a firm anterior corset has been created, platysmal bands are gone and are extremely unlikely to recur, because the platysma is then suspended posteriorly-superiorly to the mastoid periosteum, which sharpens the cervicomental angle. Even without posterior suspension, there is marked improvement in the cervicomental angle and the neckline, as described by Feldman, with large skin undermining and corset platysmaplasty (**Figs. 11** and **12**). Before using the Kelly clamp anterior platysmaplasty imbrications technique

Fig. 9. In order to create a better cervicomental angle than the patient had preoperatively, a wedge excision of the anterior border of the platysma muscle is performed for as much as 1 to 3 cm at the cervicomental angle. (*Courtesy of* Trustees of Indiana University, Indianapolis, IN, USA.)

with the corset sling suspension in my facelifting, I was doing a submentoplasty tuck-up in 12% to 15% of my facelift cases. Since I have been using this technique, I have reduced my submental tuck-up rate to 3% to 4% of all facelifts I have performed over the last 15 years. It is a proven technique that works and provides a long-lasting neckline. Measurements of the cervicomental angle improvement, both initially and at 1 year, 3 years, 10 years, and 15 years, have shown maintenance of the improved cervicomental angle despite some recurrent laxity of skin and occasional platysma muscle.[10–24]

Question 2: A moderately overweight patient desires a lower face and neck lift. The patient has no intention of losing weight. Will you offer this patient surgery, and why or why not? What is your approach to the heavy face and neck and how do you counsel this patient?

TRUSWELL

My ideal female facelift patient would be slender; of normal weight; with a long, flexible neck; strong facial bone structure; with high cheeks and a chin that is neither retrusive nor protruding. Her face would be free of heavy rhytides, marked photodamage, and overly deep nasolabial folds. The hyoid bone would be neither forward nor low in the neck. The submandibular glands would rest above the lower mandibular border. She would

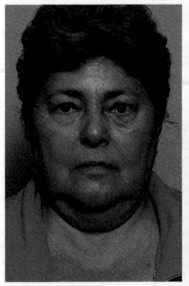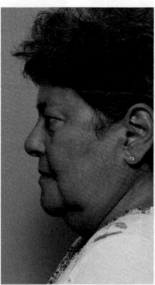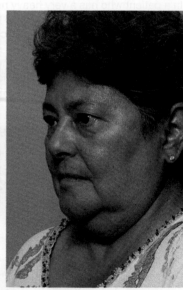

Fig. 10. In a patient who has a very heavy neck, such as a man, or in a patient with overly fatty tissues, the 3-0 Vicryl sutures are supported with 3-0 permanent braided suture, such as Mersilene. (*Courtesy of* Ethicon, Inc, Somerville, NJ.)

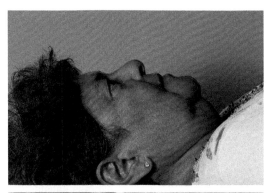

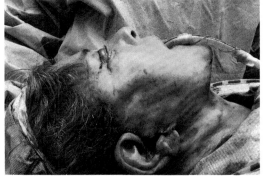

Fig. 11. Preoperative and postoperative views of a patient with a heavy neck (type III facelift patient) after a firm anterior corset has been created. This corset sharpens the cervicomental angle.

be a nonsmoker. Her goal should be to look refreshed, rejuvenated, and refeminized in an age-appropriate fashion. This ideal, alas, is not the case. Facial plastic surgeons encounter every shape and form possible in the human species.

A great challenge in facial aesthetic surgery is to recognize patients who are on the continuum of less-than-realistic expectations to outright body dysmorphia. The latter is often easier to recognize than the former. All aesthetic surgeons, at one point in their practices, have operated on patients in whom they failed to identify unrealistic expectations. As their professional lives lengthen, surgeons become more adroit in recognizing these individuals.[1,25]

One of the tenets for my practice is the great importance of patient education. Everyone in my practice plays a small to large role in educating the patient. Before I see the patient, either my practice manager or nurse greets and photographs the patient. While doing so, they conduct a friendly and informal interview to discover what are the patient's goals and desires.

They then give me a brief assessment of what to expect. I spend 45 to 60 minutes in an aging face consultation. While I chat with the patient, I can do a visual and psychological assessment.

One cohort of patients consists of people who are overweight with moderate to significantly heavy faces and necks. These individuals need counseling beyond the routine patients with aging faces.

We also encounter patients who are just too obese to undergo surgery. They pose a greater anesthesia risk. The amount of weight they would need to lose to become acceptable candidates is often beyond their capacity to achieve (**Fig. 13**).

Another set of patients present as overweight with varying degrees of fullness in the face and neck. Those with moderate fullness often have desirable results (**Figs. 14** and **15**). I always go through my full aging face consultation and then ask whether they are planning to lose weight. Most admit that they are "always" planning. For those who are sincere in losing weight, my rule of

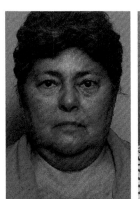
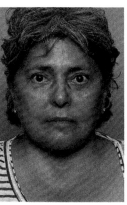
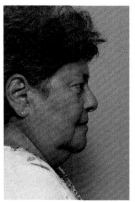
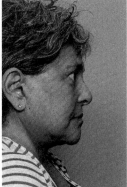

Fig. 12. Again, preoperative and postoperative views of a patient with a heavy neck after rhytidectomy. The platysmal bands are gone and are extremely unlikely to recur, because the platysma has been suspended posteriorly-superiorly to the mastoid periosteum.

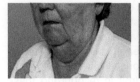
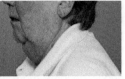

Fig. 13. This patient shows a configuration of anatomy and obesity that would not lend itself to a satisfactory outcome without considerable weight loss.

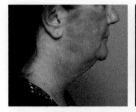
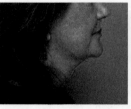

Fig. 15. Before (*left*) and after (*right*) views of a patient with a moderately heavy and full face and neck who did not wish to reduce.

thumb is for them to get within 4.5 to 7 kg (10–15 pounds) of their goals and return for further discussion. Many patients succeed in reaching their goals and return for surgery (**Fig. 16**). Some return and tell me they have lost as much as they can or that they just cannot (or will not) reduce. If I think that I can achieve sufficient improvement for them, I make certain they understand that, if we proceed and after surgery they do lose weight, then a revision is more than likely to be needed. This last group of patients need to understand that the goal is an improvement in appearance. We cannot achieve results for them that we can in a patient of normal weight with little or no facial and cervical fat. They need to understand that recurrence of jowls and wattles occurs earlier in people of heavier physiognomies and a tuck-up procedure will be needed for them earlier as well. Reaching a rapport with these patients not just on the part of the facial plastic surgeon but the whole office staff and surgical team produces acceptable results and happy outcomes (**Fig. 17**).

PUTMAN

The answer to this question is a qualified "Yes." I start the conversation by conveying a realistic expectation of results that can be achieved from facelift surgery, including adjunctive liposuction in overweight patients. I have found that before and after photographs of patients with very similar facial bone structure, habitus, sex, and age group to be invaluable in this regard. Should patient expectations not be satisfied at the end of this discussion, then I advise against any procedure.

However, should the patient express satisfaction with these results and I think that they display realistic expectations, then I proceed with the surgery.

My approach to the heavy face and neck includes full-neck tumescent liposuction and microliposuction of the jowls on many occasions. This stage is followed by a deep plane approach in most cases. The neck is approached first with submentoplasty, including subplatysmal fat sculpting and midline platysma plication with a horizontal back cut for 2 to 3 cm at the level of the hyoid bone or mentocervical break.[26] At times, I perform reduction or plication of the anterior digastric muscles. Chin augmentation is performed for all patients with significant retrognathia or prejowl sulcus recession, using the appropriate anatomic style or prejowl sulcus resection, using the appropriate anatomic style or prejowl style implant. I do not perform submandibular gland reduction but may use a Giampapa style sling or suture for selected patients with a very low hyoid bone or mentocervical break.[27,28]

Fig. 18 shows a patient with a heavy face and neck following the approach outlined earlier. No chin augmentation was performed.

PERKINS

Patients who are significantly overweight may not be candidates for facelift surgery. However, it is all relative in terms of the usual and expected status of their weight. A patient who plans a dramatic weight loss in the ensuing 3 to 6 months with rapid weight loss, such as 14 to 28 kg (30–60 pounds), should be counseled to lose most of that weight

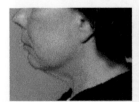
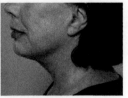

Fig. 14. Before (*left*) and after (*right*) views of a moderately heavy and full face and neck in a patient who lost 4.5 kg (10 pounds) before surgery and had no determination to lose more.

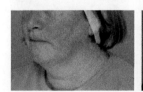
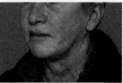

Fig. 16. Before (*left*) and after (*right*) views of a patient with a very heavy and full face and neck who lost a significant amount before surgery.

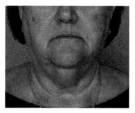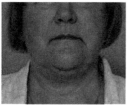

Fig. 17. Before (*left*) and after (*right*) views of a patient with a significantly heavy face and neck who had no intention of losing weight.

before having facelift surgery. Any patient who is within 7 to 9 kg (15–20 pounds) of their preoperative weight can have a satisfactory and gratifying result from facelift and neck lift surgery without affecting the overall results of the procedure, even if they continue to lose a few more kilograms. Obesity is not a contraindication to facelift and neck lift surgery, although the results of the procedure may be less than satisfactory, especially for moderately overweight patients who have no real intention to lose, or likelihood of losing, weight. It is all about managing expectations and palpating their preoperative anatomy underneath their heavy jowls and neck and lipoptosis. If the patient has a low hyoid, the expectation for a sharp neckline is diminished by preoperative consultation and visualization in front of the mirror and also with the use of computer video imaging simulation. This consultation can show patients the neckline results they can expect and also the

desired improvements can be realistic. A heavy neck can often be managed better than heavy jowls. Contouring the neck with fat sculpting, primarily using liposuction, in combination with anterior imbrications platysmaplasty and some subplatysmal fat excision, can create surprisingly good necklines in patients who otherwise look overweight. Dramatic results initially tend to relapse somewhat and patients may have a higher expectation of it needing a tuck-up procedure, if they desire, to maintain a longer lasting smoothness to the submental neckline. In consultation, in front of the mirror, I palpate the patient's soft tissues and the thickness that exists. I palpate the anatomic cervicomental angle and show the patient that everything that I can pinch between my fingers can go away, resulting in markedly improved lateral and three-quarter views of the neckline. In patients who are moderately overweight and have heavy jowls, longevity of the neckline, and particularly the jawline, can be improved by augmenting the prejowl sulcus. There may be a preexisting significant prejowl sulcus and, when lifting the cheek tissues, the surgeon can show to the patient the remaining curvilinear nature of the chin/jawline. If the chin is hypoplastic, chin augmentation provides a stronger structural basis for tightening the soft tissues and maintaining a longer lasting result. A prejowl implant is a great adjunct in maintaining a smoother jawline, even in patients with heavy cheeks and jowls, and I recommend it frequently (**Fig. 19**).

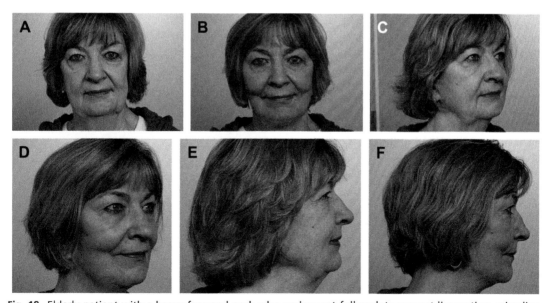

Fig. 18. Elderly patient with a heavy face and neck who underwent full-neck tumescent liposuction, microliposuction of the jowls, submentoplasty with fat sculpting, digastric muscle plication, corset platysmaplasty, and vectored extended SMAS facelift. (*A, C, E*) Preoperative views. (*B, D, F*) One-year postoperative views.

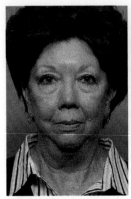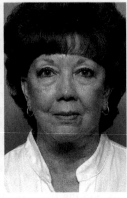

Fig. 19. A prejowl implant used as an adjunct in rhytidectomy helps maintain a smooth jawline.

Question 3: What is your mainstay procedure for repositioning the superficial musculoaponeurotic system and how, if at all, do you vary your approach?

TRUSWELL

My standard handling of the lateral SMAS follows my submental procedures. I start with a horizontal incision within the tuft of hair in front and above the auricle on the right side. Through this incision, I elevate the cheek and neck skin with progressively longer facelift scissors. I then make the posterior superior incision above the junction of the posterior edge of the auricle and the hairline. This cut extends backward into the hair and curves downward at its end. The length of this incision varies with the redundancy of the cervical skin in any given patient. Similarly, I elevate the postauricular and neck skin with blunt scissor dissection. I complete the incision around the ear at the junction of the superior helical skin and the cheek skin. It then courses just over the edge of the tragus, continues in the prelobular and postlobular creases, and courses onto the auricle over the concha joining the anterior end of the posterior superior cut.

My assistant lifts flaps with bear claw retractors. I enter beneath the SMAS at the superior edge of the tragus and elevate over the partideomasseteric fascia to just short of the anterior edge of the parotid gland with blunt scissor dissection. The elevation continues across the mandible and beneath the posterior edge of the platysma muscle downwards 3 to 4 cm. I continue the subplatysma dissection forward for about 3 cm. Last, I use the scissors to cut the SMAS flap at its superior end just below the zygoma. I continue the SMAS elevation forward to release the zygomatic cutaneous ligament (McGregor patch). I continue downward exposing the masseter muscle and inferiorly to release the mandibular cutaneous ligaments.

Once SMAS elevation is complete, I divide it into 2 flaps, cheek and cervical, at the mandible. I lift and rotate the lower corner of the cheek flap, pulling it superiorly, with tension, and tack it to the fascia at the top of the tragus (**Figs. 20** and **21**) with one 4-0 polyglactin 910 suture. The redundant superior SMAS is then removed. The cervical flap is then rotated superiorly behind the auricle with tension and tacked with one 4-0 polyglactin 910 suture to the mastoid fascia (see **Fig. 21**). Starting anterior-superiorly, I suture the entire SMAS flaps in place with a running with 2-0 PDO Quill barbed absorbable suture (Angiotech Pharmaceuticals, Vancouver, Canada). This double-armed suture is thus double sewn (**Fig. 22**).

Having performed facelift for more than 40 years, I have tried numerous techniques and variations. This sub-SMAS imbrication has been my go-to procedure for at least 20 years.

If I am doing a minilift on a thin, young woman or a tuck-up for minimal recurrence of laxity, I occasional use simple plication. I have used an SMAS-ectomy on occasion but never found it as reliable as described earlier. In my hands, this operation has produced reliable, lasting, and reproducible results.[29–31]

PUTMAN

Whether performing an extended SMAS procedure or a deep plane technique, I usually place several key vertical vectoring sutures after completely releasing all of the retaining ligaments of the face and mandible, as well as the

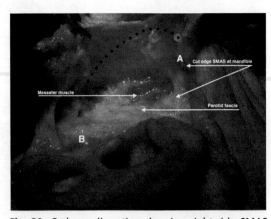

Fig. 20. Cadaver dissection showing right-side SMAS elevation over the parotid fascia exposing the masseter muscle anteriorly under its investing fascia. The SMAS has been transected at the level of the angle of the mandible. Point A will be pulled with tension and suspended at point B. The dotted line represents the approximate amount SMAS that will be resected.

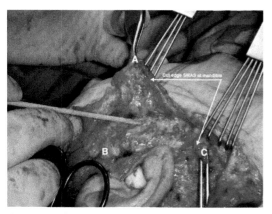

Fig. 21. Cadaver dissection showing the transected SMAS at the level of the angle of the mandible. Point A will be pulled with tension and suspended at point B. Point C is will be pulled with tension and suspended to the mastoid fascia. The pointer indicates the masseter muscle.

sternocleidomastoid cervical retaining ligaments. The first suture suspends the superior margin of the jowl firmly to the zygomatic arch periosteum. The second suture suspends the superior margin of the malar pad to deep temporal fascia. This stage is performed symmetrically. The optimal vector is determined by forceps manipulation and visual confirmation before placing the anchoring sutures and tying these down. Two or more additional vectoring sutures are then placed to suspend the inferior SMAS platysma flap to the postauricular mastoid periosteum for final repositioning of the neck tissues, but only after first repositioning the midface and jowl structures. In addition, a complete smooth SMAS closure is performed continually from the face to the neck with a

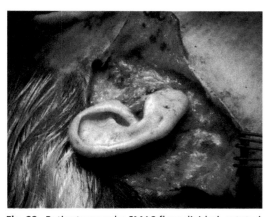

Fig. 22. Patient example: SMAS flaps divided, rotated, and imbricated with 2-0 PDO Quill barbed absorbable suture. The skin flaps have been trimmed before closure. (Available at: http://www.angiotech.com.)

running locking suture after trimming any redundant SMAS. In thin faces, I add volume by overlapping the SMAS flap in the upper face. If the SMAS is thin, weak, or attenuated, I use multiple interrupted sutures to complete the closure.[32] In addition, the platysma closure in the neck is extended about 6 cm inferior to the angle of the mandible, suturing to the sternocleidomastoid fascia primarily. I usually use a 3-0 absorbable polyglactin suture or a 2-0 PDS barbed self-locking suture for this closure. These steps are illustrated in **Figs. 23–26**.

PERKINS

The treatment of the SMAS in my routine and preferred method of rhytidectomy is extended deep plane SMAS elevation with dual-vector suspension and imbrications to create the longest lasting result in the cheek, and particularly the neckline. This technique is one that I evolved into, creating a scarification that is not dependent on suture suspension or other forms of suture soft tissue lifting. It is also a technique that is reliable and useful in nearly every patient who presents to me for correction of their neck and jawline. Whether a type I to a type III facelift, an extended SMAS rhytidectomy with deep plane elevation immobilization of the SMAS gives the patient the longest lasting result compared with other more modified or limited procedures (**Figs. 27–29**). Suspension of the SMAS in a primarily vertical direction in the cheek preauricular area, the slightly posterior movement, creates midface improvement and a natural look for the patient. Splitting the SMAS and platysma at the earlobe allows for a posterior superior suspension of the platysma and the corset created from the corset anterior platysmaplasty. This technique is a powerful method for sharpening the neckline.

SMAS manipulation requires proper incisions in the SMAS. The first incision starts at the lower edge of the zygoma anteriorly from the malar eminence extending posteriorly and diagonally inferiorly toward the earlobe (**Fig. 30**). This incision then continues inferiorly along and anterior to the border of the sternocleidomastoid muscle. Depending on the nature of the facelift, the surgeon must determine the degree of intervention and manipulation of the SMAS layer. Even type I facelifts usually require some degree of imbrication and deep plane dissection, depending on the need for elevation of midfacial tissues. The degree of undermining of the SMAS is related to the amount of movement the tissues allow once initial elevation of the SMAS is started. In my rhytidectomy technique, there is always some degree of undermining the SMAS to an advanced

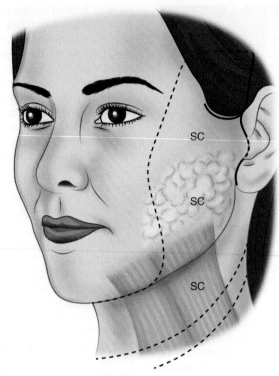

Fig. 23. Incision and subcutaneous dissection (SC).

degree of SMAS layer and platysma undermining that may be required so that it can be advanced superiorly and posteriorly at least 3 to 4 cm. The degree of this undermining is dictated by the need for lifting of the jowl and midfacial tissues; this constitutes imbrication of the SMAS, whereby the SMAS is lifted, advanced, suspended, and sutured. The variation that I use is to maintain the superior SMAS as a slip of suspension fibrotic material and not to trim it to imbricate directly to the incision line. I advance it 3 to 4 cm superiorly and slightly posteriorly and suture it to the deep postzygomatic arch tissues, and near the periosteum I do not lift it into the temporal region, nor do I suspend it to the temporalis fascia (**Fig. 31**). This technique also provides some volumization of the lateral cheek, which is often important in patients with loss of volume caused by the aging process. The suspension is done with a nonpermanent suture and is a long-term improvement because of scarification (**Fig. 32**). Permanent sutures, which in the past have extruded, are not required. However, in men with heavy soft tissues and women with heavy fatty tissues, I occasionally add a permanent suture, such as a braided Mersilene (Ethicon) suture to augment the suspension. Scarification within fat to fat layers is not predictable and may not hold or be long lasting.

I elevate the SMAS anteriorly only as far as necessary to accomplish the lift I am trying to achieve in any given patient. This elevation varies depending on the patient's individual anatomy as well as the release of the zygomatic mandibular ligament and the zygomaticus ligaments in the malar region. I only undermine this area of the malar region when I need more midfacial lifting. This undermining is done in only about 30% of my sub-SMAS dissections. Sub-SMAS dissection always extends over the fascia, covering the masseter muscle and, in about 60% of cases, involves releasing the zygomatic mandibular ligament at the McGregor patch (**Fig. 33**). When testing and moving the SMAS, the direct movement of the melolabial tissues as well as the jowl, superiorly or vertically, into a more youthful position can be seen. The SMAS is then suspended to these firm preauricular tissues at the lateral zygomatic arch as a sling suspension suture. This step is done with 0-Vicryl (Ethicon). Similarly, the SMAS is divided at the level of the earlobe (**Fig. 34**) and an inferior portion of the SMAS/platysma is sutured with an 0-Vicryl suture to the posterior mastoid periosteum, creating the supporting sling of the corset platysmaplasty (**Fig. 35**). This technique provides crisp, sharp delineation of the cervicomental angle. Any excessive adipose tissue in

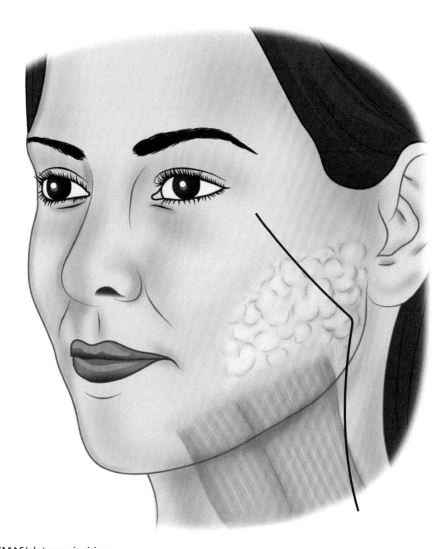

Fig. 24. SMAS/platysma incisions.

the neck is trimmed and a few sutures are placed from the suspended SMAS to the posterior post-auricular fascial soft tissues, overlapping the area of the great auricular nerve. Preauricularly, the only SMAS that is trimmed is in this region, because it is in excess. After discarding this portion of the SMAS, 3-0 Monocryl (Ethicon) sutures are used to imbricate the SMAS in the preauricular region and support the vertical suspension along the zygoma with 2 or 3 sutures placed anterior to the 0-Vicryl (Ethicon) suspension. The superior edge of the SMAS is therefore supported along the inferior border of the zygoma; this is the definition of vertical SMAS suspension with sling suspension platysmaplasty. This technique creates the most conducive situation for a natural result for the patient. Skin was elevated initially, at least 4 to 10 cm in the preauricular and premandibular region

per the markings made preoperatively in order to allow the skin to be redraped in different vectors (**Fig. 36**). This technique creates a natural, more posterior direction of the skin lift in the cheek and a superior direction in the postauricular region. This dual-vector SMAS and separate vector skin is how the preauricular hairline is managed so as not to move the anterior preauricular hair tuft, as well as to realign the posterior hairline and not have any step-off deformities.

Question 4: A patient with moderate jowl and wattle formation desires a facelift. This patient also has marked sunken cheeks. What is your recommendation for rejuvenation of the lower face and neck in this patient? If you recommend an ancillary procedure and the patient refuses and only wants the facelift, would you proceed? If so, why? If not, why not?

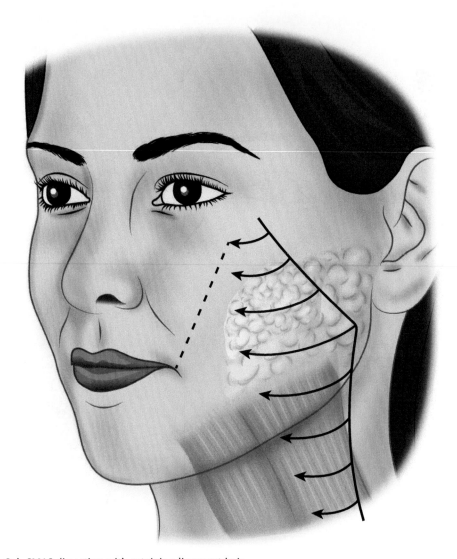

Fig. 25. Sub-SMAS dissection with retaining ligament lysis.

TRUSWELL

The face ages in 3 ways. The first signs of aging begin to appear in the mid-30s. The stratum corneum becomes adherent and the so-called glow of youth fades. Fine lines begin to appear and evidence of sun damage may become apparent. In the fifth decade, facial soft tissues begin their descent. As the decades accumulate, volume is lost in all the tissues of the face: the skin, the muscles, the fat. Even the bones of the facial skeleton change. The orbits elongate. The triangular opening of the nose flattens. If teeth are lost, the mandibular and maxillary alveolus thins down. **Fig. 37** shows the skeletal changes from infancy through adulthood to senescence.

Volume loss in the face occurs in some naturally very lean individuals and in others through the aging process. The lower cheeks and temples gain a hollow and collapsed appearance. In youth, the central portion of the face describes a circle. When people encounter a stranger, the eye picks up that circle and immediately recognizes youth before the facial appearance, manner of speech and body language, dress and so on are taken in. In more mature individuals, the circle shape transforms into an oval and the human eye instantaneously sees that stranger as older (**Fig. 38**).

When doing a consultation with a new patient who is seeking a facelift, I routinely discuss with them the 3 ways the face ages. Together we look at her face in a mirror and in my imaging program. I then discuss all signs of aging on her face. When

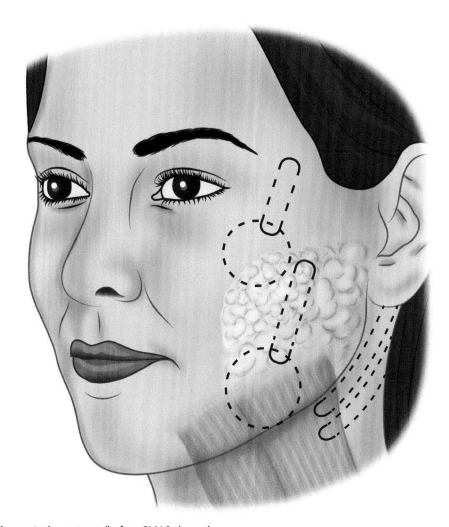

Fig. 26. Key vectoring sutures (before SMAS closure).

volume loss is small, I use minimal enhancement with one of the denser hyaluronic acid or hydroxy-apatite preparations along the malar eminence (**Fig. 39**). If the volume loss is moderate, involving the temples and upper and lower cheeks, I prefer poly-L-lactic acid (**Fig. 40**). If cheek collapse is significant, I recommend a solid silicone rubber malar, submalar, or combined cheek implant (**Fig. 41**).[33–36]

In my opinion, if a patient has numerous signs of facial aging from the forehead to the wattles, and skin, and only wishes to have a facelift or can only afford 1 operation, I am happy to agree. In consultation, I would have talked about all that I see. I do computer imaging so the patient can visualize changes and understand how a combination of procedures may be the ideal approach. If the patient understands the process and accepts softening only part of the face I will help her. Of all that clinicians can

now offer patients, a facelift alone gives an excellent outcome.

PUTMAN

Once again, I would start with patient education and realistic expectations and using before-and-after photographs of patients with similar facial habitus, sex, and age. I would be inclined to recommend a deep plane technique in this case to optimize midface improvement as well as fat transfer or even submalar implants if there is skeletal deficiency. If the patient refuses additional procedures for midface augmentation and accepts the anticipated results without hesitation, then I would proceed as outlined earlier with the understanding that additional volumizing procedures can always be performed at a later time. If the patient is at all hesitant, I would advise against surgery and suggest a second opinion or no surgery at all.

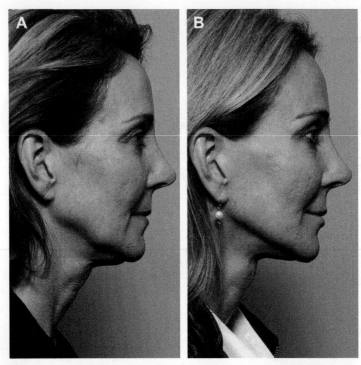

Fig. 27. Type I facelift with an extended SMAS rhytidectomy with deep plane elevation and immobilization of the SMAS gives the patient the longest lasting result compared with other more modified or limited procedures.

PERKINS

First and foremost, a facelift procedure done with the extended SMAS imbrications rhytidectomy provides a reliable and effective way to improve jowling and wattle formation. This procedure is done in combination with an anterior imbrication clamp corset platysmaplasty technique. If the patient has significant midfacial soft tissue atrophy or deficiency of bony structure, lifting the jowl and sagging midfacial tissues only partially improves the hollowness. The vertical suspension of the SMAS creates increased volumization of the

midface in many patients but has limits as to repositioning soft tissue that has aged and shown volume loss if there exists a deficient maxillary bony structure. One technique that is a long-lasting adjunctive procedure to enhancing facial volumization for facelifting is submalar/malar and mid-cheek nonautologous implant augmentation. Most patients do not require malar augmentation but, if the malar bones are hypoplastic, it will enhance the overall results of the cheek lift if a malar implant is placed. Most patients in the aging population have soft tissue volume loss, and a well-designed submalar implant placed through a small sublabial incision is an ideal adjunct to give immediate and long-lasting volumization (**Fig. 42**). These implants are generally Silastic (Dow Corning, Auburn, MI). There is a combined malar/submalar implant if both require enhancement or augmentation. The medial cheek can be augmented at the same time, placing 2-mm to 3-mm thickness Gore-Tex sheeting (expanded polytetrafluoroethylene) (WL Gore & Associates Inc, Flagstaff, AZ) medial to the infraorbital nerve to add to the submalar Silastic implant. The Silastic implant is fixated in placed anteriorly-inferiorly with a 6-mm titanium screw. Some patients prefer not to have a permanent implant in place, in which case other methods of augmentation of the midfacial bony and soft tissue are

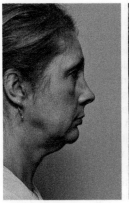
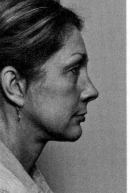

Fig. 28. Type II facelift.

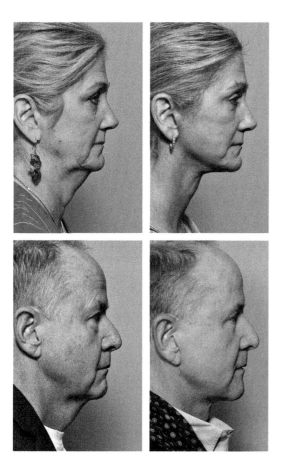

Fig. 29. (A) Type III facelift in a female patient. (B) Type III facelift in a male patient.

offered that can enhance the facelift result substantially. Easily obtained and purchased synthetic injectable material, such as hypercrosslinked hyaluronic acid, can be used to fill the midcheek malar area and submalar hollow. A variety of injectable materials are available that last from 1 to 2 years,

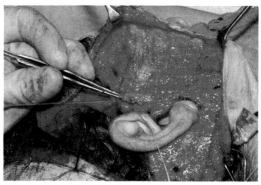

Fig. 31. The SMAS flap is advanced 3 to 4 cm superiorly and slightly posteriorly and sutured to the deep postzygomatic arch tissues near the periosteum. The flap is not lifted into the temporal region, nor is it suspended to the temporalis fascia.

or longer. Some are better for structural augmentation of the upper, middle, and malar maxilla and others are softer and are used for filling in the soft tissue hollows of the inframalar cheek. This enhancement is commonly done during rhytidectomy procedures while the patient is asleep and can be followed with office procedures, when necessary. An alternative to injectable materials is autologous fat transfer or grafting during the surgical procedure of facelifting. Fat grafting is done before the surgical facelift. The patient's own fat is obtained, either from the umbilical area, most commonly, or lateral or medial thigh. One advantage of autologous fat grafting is that it is the patient's own material and has up to a 50% chance of surviving for a 2-year period. Further fat grafting can be done as secondary procedures. However, fat grafting requires anesthesia, some degree of additional surgery, and a donor site. Compared with injectable fillers, fat

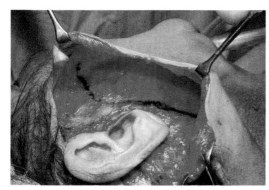

Fig. 30. The first incision of the SMAS flap starts at the lower edge of the zygoma anteriorly from the malar eminence extending posteriorly and diagonally inferiorly toward the earlobe.

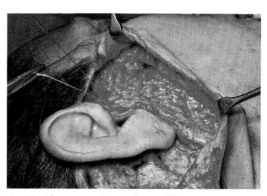

Fig. 32. The suspension is done with a nonpermanent suture and provides the patient with a long-term improvement because of scarification of the SMAS flap.

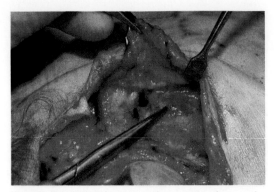

Fig. 33. Sub-SMAS dissection always extends over the fascia covering the masseter muscle and, in about 60% of cases, involves releasing the zygomatic mandibular ligament at the McGregor patch.

grafting is more expensive because of the need for an operative setting. Fat grafting is more unpredictable and various treatments with fat have been tried, with no standardized method to ensure the longest lasting volume replacement to be expected.

One additional surgical procedure used in 5% to 6% of my facelift patients is midfacelifting. Midfacelifting is a different procedure and an adjunctive procedure to replacing volume that has descended or fallen from the midfacial tissues, elongating the lower eyelid/midcheek junction. As long as the patient has volume in the lower cheek and melolabial area, midfacelifting can restore the volume in the midcheek and provide a much more youthful, long-lasting effect. This is a subperiosteal procedure that is performed in continuity with a transcutaneous lower lid blepharoplasty and temporal lift.

In addition, there are patients who, despite the definitive need for volumization of the midcheek, do not desire replacement volume or volume

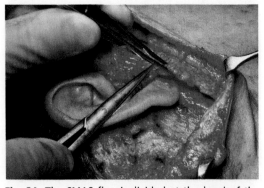

Fig. 34. The SMAS flap is divided at the level of the earlobe to allow suspension without overlap. The excess flap is trimmed as necessary.

they never had in the midcheek region. They like the way they look but are just bothered by their sagging jawlines and necklines and want to limit their surgical procedures to those areas alone. I would proceed with rhytidectomy, knowing that I can achieve their desired outcome in the neck and jawline, even if I think, aesthetically, that they should have volume to the midcheek. Some thin patients are thin all over and filling their cheeks would make them look different than they have looked and that is usually not the desire of the patient. Most patients want to look like themselves, just without the sagging jawline and neckline.

Question 5: What do you consider a successful outcome in facial rejuvenation? From "Hello" to "Goodbye", and technique aside, what is your philosophy on communicating with and educating your patients that contributes to a successful outcome?

TRUSWELL

Simply stated, a successful outcome in facial rejuvenation is a happy patient. If a patient is unhappy but the result is excellent in the surgeon's eyes, the outcome is not successful. If the patient is happy, but the surgeon is disappointed that the result is less than was wanted, the outcome is successful. When both surgeon and patient are happy, the outcome is a "homerun."

Between "Hello" and "Goodbye" there is an intricate and complicated interplay of the surgeon, nurses, office staff, physical settings, and the patient that shapes the experience and outcome of each facelift performed. The tone of things to come is set by the person who answers the office telephone. This individual must have excellent people skills. The phone should be answered within 2 rings. If the receptionist is on another line, the receptionist should politely ask whether that caller could hold for a second and wait for a response, then answer the new caller and ask that person whether she could wait for a moment and again wait for a response. It is rude to say, "Dr Jones' office could you hold" and immediately push the button. It is also rude to let the incoming call ring for several rings before answering. The receptionist must be able to answer simple questions about the doctor's credentials and the procedures performed. Clinical issues must be triaged to clinical personnel. The receptionist must always be cheerful and have an inviting mien.

The office setting should be warm and inviting. Avoid a clinical appearance. Our wafting room looks like a private club sitting room with upholstered chairs and ample art work. The clinical

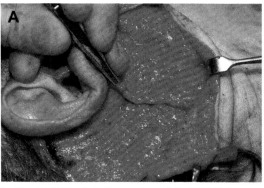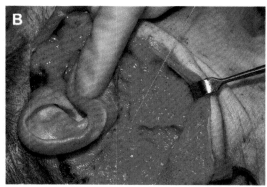

Fig. 35. (*A, B*) The inferior portion of the SMAS/platysma is sutured with an 0-Vicryl suture to the posterior mastoid periosteum, creating the supporting sling of the corset platysmaplasty. (*Courtesy of* Ethicon, Inc, Somerville, NJ.)

rooms and the aesthetic rooms are apart. The atmosphere is meant to be pleasant and unlike doctors' offices.

All staff members must have excellent people skills. Each patient should be treated as if she were warmly welcome. Many patients find multi-page intake forms annoying. Necessary information should be no more than 2 pages. Once the form is filled, the patient coordinator or office manager should quickly welcome her again and bring her to the next event in the doctor's office.

In my practice, my office manager does this and brings the patient to our photography room. She chats with the patient, eliciting as best as possible her concerns. I think a little chitchat is helpful in letting the patient feel comfortable, and this can be done during the photography process. Before bringing the patient to meet me, my officer manager gives me the new chart and her insights from conversing with the patient.

I greet the patient in my own office for the consultation. Opposite my desk is a sofa and armchair grouped facing a monitor screen. I spend a few moments talking with the patient to get to know her. Pleasantries aside, I ask what she would like to

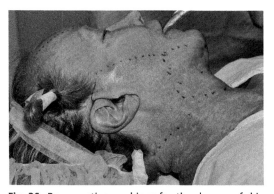

Fig. 36. Preoperative markings for the degree of skin undermining in a typical facelift.

talk with me about. I tailor my remarks based on her comments. I describe briefly how the face ages and bring her images up on the monitor. I want to know whether she only wants to hear about 1 specific issue or her face in general. I illustrate my discussion while imaging her pictures. Then I show her examples of my patients who had facelifts. During the consultation, I inform her that the procedure is done in my accredited operating room. I describe the anesthesia used and the perioperative experience. During this interview, I assess her for realistic expectations and ascertain whether she is a good candidate for a facelift.

Once all questions and concerns have been addressed, my office manager discusses pricing and scheduling with her. Three weeks before surgery, the patient returns to meet with a nurse for preoperative instructions. The nurse reiterates the entire perioperative experience. If the patient wants to ask me more questions at this time, I am available. I, my nurses, and my office manager all stress throughout the process that part of a good outcome is the patient understanding her responsibilities, which includes understanding what will occur and what she must do preoperatively and postoperatively. This requirement is reiterated to her on all encounters.

On the day of surgery, the patient changes in a side room. I mark the patient and anesthesia interviews her outside the surgical suite. In the operating room, music is playing softly. Anesthesia starts the intravenous line and gently induces sedation. Recovery is smooth and quick, and the patient is discharged when alert and has eaten and had something to drink. The patient is called the evening of surgery. The next day, the dressing is removed and the nurse washes and blow-dries the patient's hair. The postoperative instructions are reviewed again with me and the nurse. We usually see the patient a few days later and again on day 8. The patient returns in 6 to 8 weeks for

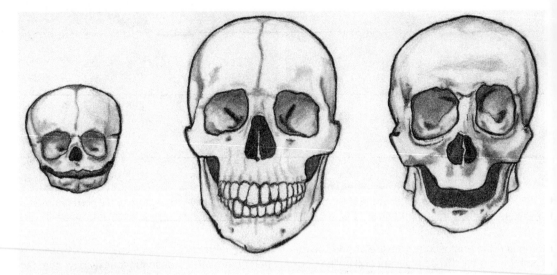

Fig. 37. Artist's depiction of the changes of the human facial skeleton from infancy (*left*) through middle age (*middle*) to senescence (*right*). (*Courtesy of* Jason Truswell, Charleston, SC.)

a cosmetic makeover and photographs. At this time, an aesthetician talks with the patient about ongoing skin care and arranges to see her periodically for light chemical peels.

Every step of the way, we try to make the patient feel cared for and cared about. My entire staff is dedicated to the nurturing ideal of the practice. We want patients to return and wish them to speak highly of us and our services.

PUTMAN

Aesthetic facial surgery is a quality-of-life specialty in which the satisfaction of the patient may be the most important outcome metric. Therefore, understanding the factors that influence the patient's satisfaction is integral for maintaining a successful practice. Although functional and reconstructive procedures can

use easily measurable parameters, aesthetic procedures must be measured in terms of how the patient feels about the procedures that have affected their appearance. From both a philosophic and practical standpoint, I try to emphasize the importance of a natural-looking outcome to the patient. In this regard, I still use patient photographs from their younger years as an adjunct to identify the aging face changes that have occurred and that are amenable to treatment with aesthetic surgery and other procedures. Most patients just want to look like a younger version of themselves.

This being the case, the next essential is conveying reasonable expectations regarding the surgical outcome to the patient through consultation. In addition, the success of the overall journey from initial consultation, preoperative planning and preparation, through the surgical encounter and

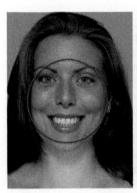
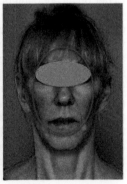

Fig. 38. (*Left*) The circle of a youthful face. (*Right*) The oval in a very slim face.

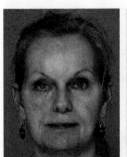
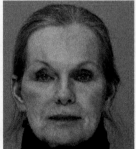

Fig. 39. A 65-year-old patient before (*left*) and after (*right*) volume enhancement with Restylane Lyft in the midface. (Available at: www.galdermausa.com.)

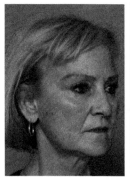
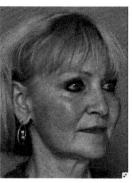

Fig. 40. A 66-year-old before (*left*) and after (*right*) 4 series of injections of Sculptra in the temples, upper cheeks, and lower cheeks. (Available at: http://www.angiotech.com.)

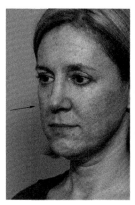
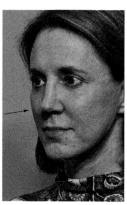

Fig. 42. A well-designed submalar implant placed through a small sublabial incision (*arrows*) is an ideal adjunct to give immediate and long-lasting volumization.

recovery must all be considered in the light of an established trusted relationship in which the surgeon's commitment to the patient is without question.

PERKINS

A successful outcome in facial rejuvenation is the result of applying a time-proven technique to each unique and individual patient. The key is applying time-proven surgical techniques that work and last. Trying to minimize the procedure and limit its scope results in a minimal result and a limited and unsatisfactory outcome over the longer term. Patients are interested in having a result, but would love the surgeon to tell them that it only takes this small amount of surgery or even a nonsurgical approach in order to achieve the result. Being honest with patients in the initial consultation and not succumbing to their fears but guiding them to understand that what it takes to achieve their desired results is often surgical intervention that works on a long-term basis. A natural and long-lasting result that minimizes complication is the goal of facial rejuvenation surgery (**Fig. 43**). A natural look is what patients are looking for. Many are so afraid because of what they have seen in photographs of celebrities or

celebrities themselves who supposedly had the ability to choose the best surgeons possible. They do not want a pulled look and they do not want to look like someone else. They want to be rejuvenated and just want to look like themselves when they were younger. Most patients do not even want anyone to realize they have had a facelift. They just want to look refreshed and rested, with a prettier (more youthful) neckline. So, when surgical techniques can be applied to achieve those goals, the result is a happy patient population, a satisfied surgeon, and a gratifying doctor-patient experience (**Figs. 44** and **45**).

It is vital that the patient be medically stable and healthy before the procedure, because this is cosmetic surgery and there are patients who are not candidates to undergo a proper facelift. It is equally important that the patient has proper psychological and emotionally stability, with realistic expectations, to tolerate the initial postoperative healing time and course. Patients must understand and be prepared to accept that the surgery has its own inherent postoperative issues that take time to resolve in order to achieve the final desired result.

Communicating the limitations and potential complications of the surgery is critical to ensure reasonable patient expectations. Most of this is established during the initial consultation but these issues need to be reiterated throughout the preoperative planning and the immediate and continued postoperative course. Studies have shown that patients only retain approximately 8% of what they were told during the initial consultation, whether the consultation was 10 minutes or 1 hour in length. I spend 30 to 40 minutes with each patient with an aging face, depending on the number of procedures desired. The patient is

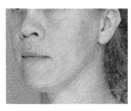
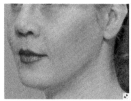

Fig. 41. A 30-year-old patient before (*left*) and after (*right*) solid silicon rubber submalar implants in both cheeks.

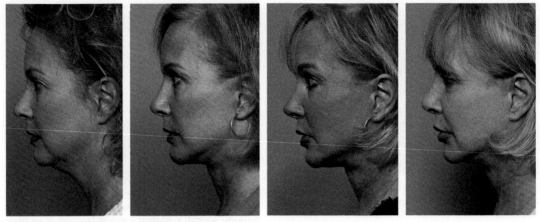

Fig. 43. Type I facelift result over 13 years.

in my office a minimum of 1.5 hours. When the patient first calls to request a consultation, it is imperative that the office person who answers the phone is knowledgeable, warm, and receptive. This person may be able to provide enough information but I do not think it is appropriate to quote prices on the phone, other than general ranges. Each patient presents with a unique set of issues in rejuvenation surgery and front reception personnel cannot be expected to specify the cost of rejuvenation without the doctor having examined the patient. Once patients initially come to the office, they are first met by a photographer who takes preoperative photographs. The photographer also asks what procedures they are interested in and proceeds to use computer simulation or computer imaging to show them what the expected results may look like. During the time of the photographer's imaging manipulation, the patient is taken into the consultation room by a physician's assistant who goes over many

medical issues and questions; talks about what will happen during the rest of the consultation and where the surgery is done; and informs them, as much as possible, about what to expect in relation to the potential of having cosmetic rejuvenation surgery.

I then meet the patient with the physician's assistant and spend 20 to 30 minutes evaluating the patient. I think it is critical, after asking about the patient's desires and understanding what bothers the patient most, to sit the patient in front of a 3-way mirror. Depending on the patient's desire for me to comment on other procedures that may enhance the overall look, I concentrate on what bothers the patient most. For rhytidectomy patients, I am able to show with my hands exactly what surgery will accomplish. It is a powerful way of looking at themselves with my hands holding their sagging, aging soft tissues back into a more youthful position. This demonstration is something that most patients do not do

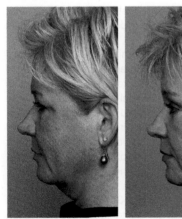
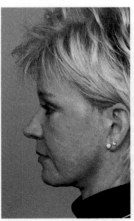
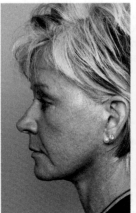
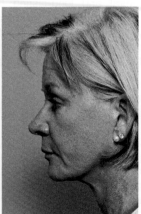

Fig. 44. Type II facelift result over 11 years.

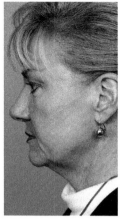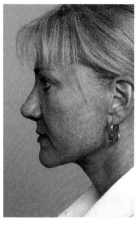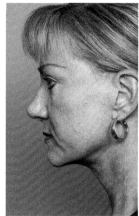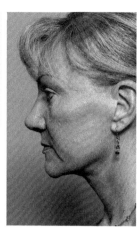

Fig. 45. Type III facelift result over 6 years.

accurately when pulling their own facial tissues upward and backward to try to see what it would look like to have a rejuvenated jawline and neckline. I also use the 3-way mirror so they can visualize their neckline structures, how they looked before surgery, and how they would look after I tighten things surgically. At this time I discuss how things are improved surgically. Even if patients come in stating they do not want a facelift, I do not let terminology determine whether or not the patient is a candidate for a facelift or neck lift only; I just show them what it takes to get the neckline/jawline they desire. If they understand that a standard rhytidectomy involves a cheek and neck lift with primary emphasis on the neck, then they are satisfied at the beginning of preoperative planning and agreement to proceed with surgery. Once patients realizes they are going to look normal and look like themselves and understand that this is a surgical procedure, I take the patient back into the photographer's room and show them the expected results on the video imaging computer. Doing this can be extremely powerful, particularly on the lateral view, which patients do not normally see. Even if they saw it in the 3-way mirror, they do not generally see it in pictures or in front of the mirror themselves. It can also visually demonstrate to the patients their limits, as well as what their underlying structure can be. The more the patients realistically see how they look in a simulation, the more comfortable they are about proceeding with surgery.

However, after the video imaging consultation and before talking to the patient care coordinator for surgical scheduling, it is extremely valuable for the patient to see true before-and-after photographs of patients who have had a similar procedure. This experience reassures them and enhances their confidence that they will look natural and like themselves and will not look like someone they can point out who looks like they have had a facelift. The more prepared the patient is before surgery regarding how much time is required to heal and be away from work and other social activities, the happier the patient is (with the experience and the outcome) and the happier the outcome. There is a prolonged healing time for rhytidectomy, most of which is sensation related and not visual. Visually, patients can reassimilate fairly quickly to their normal social and work activities but must understand that patience is required to get through the full healing process and obtain the final result 6 to 12 months postoperatively.

Question 6: How has your approach to rejuvenation of the lower face and neck changed over the last 5 years?

TRUSWELL

Over the last 5 to 10 years, I have taught my facelift patients to understand the three-dimensional way their faces age. I want them to come to know the aging process, and how the aging of the skin, the sagging of the soft tissues, and volume loss in the cheeks and temples interplay in their maturing appearance. When possible, I like to address all the aspects of the older face in their entirety. I am happiest when I can lift the ptotic brow, rejuvenate the eyelids, raise the sagging lower face and neck, restore volume, and resurface the skin. This outcome is not always possible for many reasons. Probably the greatest reason is financial concerns. In most cases the most dramatic single improvement is from a facelift.

I have shortened my posterior superior incision to about 12 mm (0.5 inch). This length is applicable in most patients. One exception is the patients with considerable redundant cervical skin that needs a great amount of redraping.

I have also started using QuikClot hemostatic dressing (Z-Medica, LLC, Wallingford, CT). I find this is a great help in controlling bleeding during the procedure and bruising afterward. Once I have created and imbricated the SMAS flaps and trimmed the skin flaps, I place a piece of the gauze on top of the SMAS. I open and roll a 4 × 4 gauze over this followed by another QuikClot gauze. The skin flaps are then put in place. After 10 minutes the flaps are lifted and the gauzes gently removed. The surgical bed is essentially completely dry. One or 2 bleeding points may be seen and are easily cauterized (**Fig. 46**).

The other change I have made is the use of 2-0 PDO Quill barbed absorbable suture (Angiotech Pharmaceuticals, Vancouver, Canada) to suture the SMAS flaps as well as imbrication of the anterior bands. The suture is double armed with the barbs pointing away from each needle to the bare midpoint of the suture. I doubly oversew the SMAS and platysma imbrications. The suture does not require tying and the barbs create a strong hold on the tissues. This method reduces closure time considerably.

PUTMAN

Over the last 5 years and more, I have become much more selective about using minilift techniques in general, reserving various short scar or plication-based procedures for younger patients, typically in their 40s, and possibly early 50s, primarily. These patients would be the type I individuals in the Perkins classification and others with good skin elasticity, minimal jowling, lipodystrophy and cheek ptosis, and thin faces. Many of these

patients can benefit from the additional volumizing afforded by plication procedures or overlapping the SMAS flap. On all other patients, I have favored a vectored extended SMAS technique as previously described, or a classic deep plane approach with vertical orientation. Along these lines, I routinely release all facial ligamentous structures, including the zygomatic masseteric, mandibular, and sternocleidomastoid cervical retaining ligaments to achieve better redraping and long-term results. This technique has reduced the need for secondary revisions such as submentoplasty considerably in my patient population. I have also stopped performing routine midlines and submental platysma plication, especially in patients who can be addressed with the more vertically oriented facelift technique described earlier.[37–47]

PERKINS

First, having been in practice for 34 years, my technique for obtaining an excellent neckline and long-lasting result of the neckline and jawline in rhytidectomy has not changed substantially in the last 5 years. However, it has been substantially modified and has become a bit more aggressive in the surgical approach than when I first started practice. In the first 5 years of practice, I was primarily doing plication (fold-over) SMAS rhytidectomy and trying to apply this to every patient. I tried various methods of treatment of the platysma, from nonsuture imbrication to plication of the anterior borders of the platysma after posterior suspension. None of these procedure worked on most patients in the type 2 and type 3 categories. The less involved facelift of skin undermining fold-over plication with minimum neck work was effective in several type I rhytidectomy patients but failed substantially within 1 to 1.5 years in most

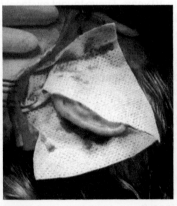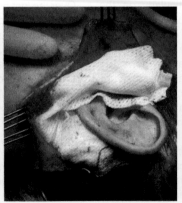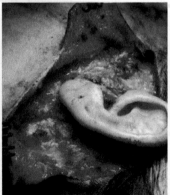

Fig. 46. (*Left*) QuikClot hemostatic dressing placed on the imbricated SMAS during a facelift. (*Center*) A second layer of QuikClot over a rolled 4 × 4 placed on the first layer. (*Right*) The surgical bed is essentially completely dry after 10 minutes. (*Courtesy of* Z-Medica, LLC, Wallingford, CT.)

advanced level type II and type III patients with heavy necks, significant waddling in the neck, lipoptosis, and heavy jowls. My technique of advancing the undermining of the SMAS and repositioning the SMAS with imbrication techniques and then sling suspension evolved over the next 10 to 15 years. Studying my own results over a 15-year period with measurements showed me that what I suspected clinically was working statistically. Doing the anterior clamp platysmaplasty corset suspension platysmaplasty was something that has long-lasting results, works better in the short term, and lasts well into the 10-year to 15-year range. Many patients never return to their preoperative conditions. In the last 5 to 7 years, improvements in the midface have been the goal in my facelift surgeries, as well as generally for most surgeons. This goal requires either midface-lifting or augmentation of the midface with techniques that last or can easily be repeated. Most significantly, the facelift technique involved a little less posterior movement of the undermined cheek SMAS and more of a vertical suspension. By lifting the midfacial tissues and keeping them in that position without trimming the SMAS and using it for volume, as well as a sling suspension, I was able to achieve the best results possible. Adding prejowl implants over the past 10 years has improved the heavy jowl and neckline for the longer term. Most importantly, reducing the need for permanent sutures or relying on sutures to hold the suspension by undermining and overlapping the SMAS has again proved to be successful, with both the patients and myself, as the surgeon, happier with the result. The degree of undermining has varied and can be aggressive, releasing the malar dermal attachments at the McGregor patch in the malar area all the way to the zygomatic mandibular ligament; it depends on the patient and the movement allowed while undermining the SMAS. It is deep plane rhytidectomy with a separate vector in undermining the skin to allow the skin and the SMAS platysma to be tightened in different directions and not simultaneously. With the superior vector of the SMAS and the posterior suspension of the corset platysmaplasty done after the anterior imbrication and tightening, I have reduced my submental tuck-up procedures from 12% to 14% to 2% to 3% of all rhytidectomies. This reduction has resulted in cost savings and a more satisfied patient population. Recurrent rebound relaxation in the submental area is natural and unavoidable in some situations but is minimized by these more aggressive approaches. Recurrent sagging of the jowl requiring cheek tuck-ups occurs in less than 2% of my patient population and is usually in patients who did not have as much vertical suspension of the SMAS or had preexisting heavy jowls. I do open liposuction to fat overlying the midcheek and jowl on heavier patients and this has improved the lasting results of the neck and jawline in these patient populations.

Reducing complications is a primary goal in any cosmetic procedure. Facelifting has a certain degree of complications, including hematoma, seroma, recurrent relaxation, and even temporary motor and neurosensory weakness. Careful selection of patients, and not operating on patients with autoimmune diseases or smokers who are recalcitrant and cannot stop smoking, has reduced any incidence of vascular compromise and skin slough. Skin slough, however, can occur but compression dressings and the use of drains in most patients is still a mainstay in my rhytidectomy patients with full neck and cheek undermining. Attempts to minimize incision length have not been found to be useful and the length of the incision to properly redrape the skin and realign the hairline have not caused any patient dissatisfaction in the short and long terms postoperatively. Therefore, I do not shorten my incisions but allow myself to perform an adequate undermining suspension and redraping for the best and maximal long-term result.

REFERENCES

1. McCullough EG, Perkins SW, Thomas R. Facelift panel discussion, controversies and techniques. Facial Plast Surg Clin North Am 2012;20(3):279–325.
2. Loyo M, Kontis TC. Cosmetic botulinum toxin: has it replaced more invasive facial procedures? Facial Plast Surg Clin North Am 2013;21(2):285–98.
3. Truswell WH. The facelift: a guide for safe, reliable, and reproducible results. In: Truswell WH, editor. Surgical facial rejuvenation a roadmap to safe and reliable outcomes. New York: Thieme Medical Publishers; 2008. p. 24–45.
4. Perkins SW, Balikian RV. Extended superficial musculoaponeurotic system (SMAS) facelift. In: Truswell WH, editor. Surgical facial rejuvenation a roadmap to safe and reliable outcomes. New York: Thieme Medical Publishers; 2008. p. 47–53.
5. Feldman JJ. Corset platysmaplasty. Plast Reconstr Surg 1990;85(3):333–43.
6. Guyuron B, Sadeck EY, Ahmadian R. A 26 year experience with vest-over-pants technique platysmarrhaphy. Plast Reconstr Surg 2010;126(3):1027–34.
7. Henly JL, Lesniak DJ, Terk AR. Contralateral platysma suspension: an adjunct to rhytidectomy. Arch Facial Plast Surg 2005;7:119–23.
8. Feldman JJ. Neck lift my way: an update. Plast Reconstr Surg 2014;134(6):1173–83.

9. Feldman JJ. Corset platysmaplasty. Clin Plast Surg 1992;19(2):369–82.

10. Skoog T. Plastic surgery: the aging face. In: Skoog TG, editor. Plastic surgery: new methods and refinements. Philadelphia: WB Saunders; 1974. p. 300–30.

11. Mitz V, Peyronnie M. The superficial musculo-aponeurotic system (SMAS) in the parotid and cheek area. Plast Reconstr Surg 1976;58:80.

12. Baker SR. Triplane rhytidectomy. Combining the best of all worlds. Arch Otolaryngol Head Neck Surg 1997;123:1167–72.

13. Adamson P, Moran ML. Complications of cervicofacial rhytidectomy. Facial Plast Surg Clin North Am 1993;112:257–70.

14. Perkins SW. Achieving the "natural look" in rhytidectomy. Facial Plast Surg 2000;16:269–82.

15. Perkins SW, Archer KA. The extended SMAS facelift. In: Constantinides M, Thomas R, Chauham N, editors. Expert techniques in facial plastic surgery: an analytical approach to facelift and necklift surgery. New Delhi (India): Jaypee Brothers Medical Publishers; 2015.

16. Perkins SW, Brobst RW. Perkins' Kelly clamp technique for submental platysmaplasty with a modified extended SMAS facelift: objective evaluation and long-term outcomes, in press.

17. Perkins SW, Waters HH. The extended SMAS approach to neck rejuvenation. Facial Plast Surg Clin North Am 2014;22(2):253–68.

18. Perkins SW, Williams JD, Macdonald K, et al. Prevention of seromas and hematomas after face-lift surgery with the use of postoperative vacuum drains. Arch Otolaryngol Head Neck Surg 1997; 123:743–5.

19. Chaffoo RA. Complications in facelift surgery: avoidance and management. Facial Plast Surg Clin North Am 2013;21:551–8.

20. Rees TD, Aston SJ. A clinical evaluation of the results of sub-musculoaponeurotic dissection and fixation in face lifts. Plast Reconstr Surg 1977;60:851.

21. Jones BM, Lo SJ. How long does a face lift last? Objective and subjective measurements over a 5-year period. Plast Reconstr Surg 2012;130:1317–27.

22. Riefkohl R, Wolfe JA, Cox EB, et al. Association between cutaneous occlusive vascular disease, cigarette smoking, and slough after rhytidectomy. Plast Reconstr Surg 1986;77:592–5.

23. Kamer F. Sequential rhytidectomy and the two-stage concept. Otolaryngol Clin North Am 1980;13:305–20.

24. Anderson JR. The tuck-up operation: a new technique of secondary rhytidectomy. In: Kaye BL, Gradinger DP, editors. Symposium on problems and complications in aesthetic plastic surgery of the face. St Louis (MO): Mosby; 1984. p. 162–70.

25. Sarwer DB, Wadden TA, Pertschuck MJ, et al. Body image dissatisfaction and body dysmorphic disorder in 100 cosmetic surgery patients. Plast Reconstr Surg 1998;101:1644–9.

26. Perkins SW, Gibson FB. Use of submentoplasty to enhance cervical recontouring in facelift surgery. Arch Otolaryngol Head Neck Surg 1993;119(2): 179–83.

27. Giampapa UC, Bernardo BE. Neck recontouring with suspension suture and liposuction. Aesthetic Plast Surg 1995;19:217–23.

28. Caplin DA, Prendiville S. Modifications in rejuvenation of the aging neck. Facial Plast Surg Clin North Am 2002;10(1):77–86.

29. Perkins SW, Dayan S. Rhytidectomy. In: Papel I, editor. Facial plastic and reconstructive surgery. 2nd edition. New York: Thieme Medical Publishers; 2002. p. 153–70.

30. Larrabee WF, Makielski KH, Henderson JL. Surgical anatomy of the face. 2nd edition. Philadelphia: Lippincott Williams & Wilkins; 2004.

31. Becker FF, Bassichis BA. Deep plane face-lift vs. superficial musculoaponeurotic system plication facelift. Arch Facial Plast Surg 2004;6:8–13.

32. Beaty MM. A progressive approach to neck rejuvenation. Facial Plast Surg Clin North Am 2014;22(2): 177–90.

33. Godin M, Costa L, Romo T, et al. Gore-Tex chin implants: a review of 324 cases. Arch Facial Plast Surg 2003;5:224–7.

34. Godin M, Hamilton JS. Facial skeletal implants. In: Truswell WH, editor. Surgical facial rejuvenation a roadmap to safe and reliable outcomes. New York: Thieme Medical Publishers; 2008. p. 100–12.

35. Binder WJ. Submalar augmentation: an alternative to face-lift surgery. Arch Facial Plast Surg 1989; 115(7):797–801.

36. Binder WJ, Azizzadeh B. Malar and submalar augmentation. Facial Plast Surg Clin North Am 2008;16(1):11–32.

37. Jacono AA. Vertical neck lifting. Facial Plast Surg Clin North Am 2014;22(2):285–316.

38. Mendelson BC. Anatomic study of the retaining ligaments of the face and application for facial rejuvenation. Aesthetic Plast Surg 2013;37(3): 513–5.

39. Perkins SW, Patel AB. Extended superficial muscular aponeurotic system rhytidectomy: a graded approach. Facial Plast Surg Clin North Am 2009;17(4):575–87, vi.

40. Jacono AA, Parikh SS. The minimal access deep plane extended vertical facelift. Aesthet Surg J 2011;31(8):874–90.

41. Ellenbogen R, Karlin JV. Visual criteria for success in restoring the youthful neck. Plast Reconstr Surg 1980;66(6):826–37.

42. Hamra ST. The deep plane rhytidectomy. Plast Reconstr Surg 1990;86(1):53–61.

43. Dedo DD. "How I do it"–plastic surgery. Practical suggestions on facial plastic surgery. A

preoperative classification of the neck for cervico-facial rhytidectomy. Laryngoscope 1980;90(11 Pt 1):1894–6.

44. Marten TJ. High SMAS facelift: combined single flap lifting of the jawline, cheek and mid face. Clin Plast Surg 2008;35(4):569–603. vi-vii.

45. Shah AR, Rosenberg D. Defining the facial extent of the platysma muscle: a review of 71 consecutive face-lifts. Arch Facial Plast Surg 2009;11(6):405–8.

46. Jacono AA, Parkh SS, Kennedy WA. Anatomical comparison of platysmal tightening using superficial musculoaponeurotic system plication vs deep-plane rhytidectomy techniques. Arch Facial Plast Surg 2011;13(6):395–7.

47. Adamson PA, Dahiya R, Litner J. Midface effects of the deep-plane vs the superficial musculoaponeurotic system plication face-lift. Arch Facial Plast Surg 2007;9(1):9–11.

Facial Paralysis Discussion and Debate

Travis T. Tollefson, MD, MPH[a], Tessa A. Hadlock, MD[b], Jessyka G. Lighthall, MD[c],*

KEYWORDS

- Facial paralysis • Facial reanimation • Gracilis • Temporalis tendon transfer • Advances

KEY POINTS

- Routine assessment of the patient with facial paralysis should include a clinician-graded outcome measure, a patient-graded outcome measure, standardized photographic documentation, and videography.
- Neuromuscular retraining remains the first-line treatment for patients with synkinesis.
- The use of the masseteric branch of the trigeminal nerve as a neural source has advanced reanimation of the paralyzed face.
- Future treatments will likely involve factors to guide neural regeneration, implantable stimulators driven by the unaffected side, and a focus on quality of life improvement.

Panel discussion

1. What do you use routinely to evaluate patient outcomes and what are the benefits and limitations of these measures? What do you think the minimal assessment standards should be in evaluating results of facial reanimation procedures?

2. Are there any techniques that you have migrated away from using and what have you replaced them with? In which clinical situations would you still use these procedures?

3. What is the role of nonsurgical treatments and surgical therapies (eg, neurectomy, myectomy) in the treatment of patients with postparesis synkinesis in your practice? What are the limitations of these therapies?

4. When using free muscle transfer for reanimation, what modifications or pearls can you offer to optimize outcomes?

5. What do you see as the future of treatment for patients with facial paralysis and what are key areas where research should focus?

6. What is the single most important advancement in technique for the treatment of facial paralysis that you have adopted in the past 5 years? How else has your facial reanimation practice evolved over the past 5 years?

Disclosure Statement: The authors have nothing to disclose.
[a] Facial Plastic and Reconstructive Surgery, Department of Otolaryngology–Head and Neck Surgery, University of California, Davis, UC Davis Medical Center, 2521 Stockton Boulevard, Suite 7200, Sacramento, CA 95817, USA; [b] Division of Facial Plastic and Reconstructive Surgery, Department of Otolaryngology–Head and Neck Surgery, Massachusetts Eye and Ear Infirmary, Harvard Medical School, 243 Charles Street, Boston, MA 02114, USA; [c] Division of Otolaryngology-Head and Neck Surgery, Penn State Hershey Medical Center, 500 University Drive H-091, Hershey, PA 17033, USA
* Corresponding author.
E-mail address: jlighthall@pennstatehealth.psu.edu

Facial Plast Surg Clin N Am 26 (2018) 163–180
https://doi.org/10.1016/j.fsc.2017.12.004

Question 1: What do you use routinely to evaluate patient outcomes and what are the benefits and limitations of these measures? What do you think the minimal assessment standards should be in evaluating results of facial reanimation procedures?

TOLLEFSON

At our center, we routinely use a team-based approach to evaluation of patient outcomes. First, we use routine photograph and video analysis. Next, we collect patient reported outcome measures (PROMs). The advantage is that we evaluate comparative effectiveness using the data, and the disadvantage is that collection and cataloging this data are time and labor intensive. At a minimum, I collect the following information using instruments to account for potential gaps in the perceptions of patient, surgeon and lay public.[1] The PROMs or quality-of-life instrument that we use is the validated Facial Clinimetric Evaluation (FaCE), which captures the symptoms and impact of the facial paralysis on daily life.[2] Last, all patients are assessed with the Nasal Obstruction Symptom Evaluation scale to allow for longitudinal assessment of the nasal obstruction related to facial paralysis and external nasal valve collapse (**Fig. 1**).[3]

Relying on standardized clinical photographs of before and after treatment as a sole measure has significant limitations for facial paralysis. The dynamic aspects of patients with facial paralysis can be captured with video of spontaneous activities; however, this is difficult owing to

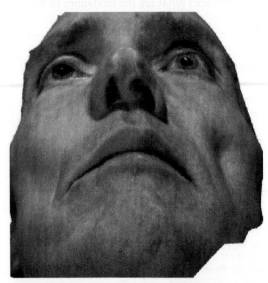

Fig. 1. Base view on 3-dimensional stereophotogrammetry demonstrating patient with right facial paralysis and columella pulled to the left with a right-sided external nasal valve collapse.

time constraints in a clinical setting. I capture the standardized photographs, including frontal, profile (left and right), oblique (left and right), and base view, while adding the following:

- Frontal with eyes closed passively,
- Frontal with eyes maximal closure, and
- Patient voicing the vowels "a," "e," and "o."

This sequence captures the excursing of the lateral commissure of the lips, the inferior lower lip pull on the nonparalyzed side and lip puckering.

In the last 2 years, I began capturing video (2–3 minutes) of the patient telling a story with spontaneous connected speech (eg, asking to discuss pets or children). I believe that this is labor intensive, but ultimately allows an assessment of how the face is emotive and unprompted. Last, for measurement of symmetry, I capture stereophotogrammetry using the VectraM3 (Canfield, Atlanta, GA). The automated analysis is helpful for general symmetry, but is most beneficial when counseling patients and discussing reasonable expectations.

HADLOCK

In my practice, we routinely use 4 types of outcome assessment tools to evaluate patients with facial paralysis, including a clinician-graded measure, a patient-graded assessment, a quantitative measure, and a lay person assessment (CPQL[Clinician-Patient-Quantitative-Layperson] model).[4,5] For clinician-graded outcomes assessment, we prefer to use the eFACE software, which was developed at Massachusetts Eye and Ear Infirmary.[6] It is a quick bedside digital platform with 15 measures (4 static, 7 dynamic, and 4 synkinesis measures) on a visual analog scale that provides an immediate graphical rendering compared with the patient's healthy side. The eFACE can be performed serially to provide a pictorial view of the patient's progress and it has been rigorously internally and externally validated with high intrarater and interrater reliability, and has good correlation with expert grading of facial disfigurement both for live patient and video assessments of function.[7,8] Additionally, we evaluated the sensitivity of the eFACE to change such that, after an intervention has been performed on a patient, it was found to have a high sensitivity for detecting that change. The eFACE program is widely available with a downloadable app with an online tutorial available for clinicians.

It is important to include a PROM in a facial nerve practice. Although many PROMs exist, we prefer the FaCE instrument.[2] This instrument has been rigorously validated in the literature and is a widely used tool.

We incorporate quantitative objective measures for outcomes using the Facial Assessment by Computer Evaluation (FACE) software to compare the affected and unaffected side.[9] Specific features we examine are smile excursion, palpebral fissure width, the number of millimeters of brow ptosis with attempted brow elevation, and the degree of symmetry of the upper and lower lip.[10] The FACE gram program allows for precise calculations based on standardized photographic views and allows for an objective measure for critically evaluating patient outcomes after treatment. We also obtain standardized videographic assessments of patients. The benefit of video documentation is that this becomes part of the patient's permanent record. As new grading scales emerge, this measure allows us to reliably compare that scale to what was previously available. In addition, some concerns arise that may only be noted on dynamic movement that would otherwise not be perceptible on still photos.

The final measure in the CPQL model is the layperson assessment. This is not quite part of our assessment battery yet, but we are actively studying ways to incorporate a layperson assessment into our model. A study is currently underway that involves showing naïve observers video clips and having them grade patients with facial weakness. Based on their responses, a disfigurement score can be obtained and provides a mathematical calculation for attractiveness based on layperson assessments. Changes in these scores over time can help to assess the recovery of facial motion after a paralysis as well as help us to evaluate the impact our treatments have on the perceived attractiveness of patients by lay persons.

At a minimum, every person who takes care of facial nerve patients should administer a PROM and a clinician-graded outcome assessment. Most people who treat facial nerve patients no longer feel that the House-Brackmann Scale is adequate to assess patients or develop management strategies. The House-Brackmann Scale was not designed to help us identify facial function in all patients. Rather, it was designed to describe recovery of the facial nerve after vestibular schwannoma surgery. The Facial Nerve Grading System 2.0 was developed in an attempt to address some of these shortcomings, although it never gained widespread adoption.[11] Multiple other clinician-graded instruments have been developed. Currently, no perfect grading system exists and providers should select a system that works well for their practice and provides segmental information, assesses synkinesis, and assists in treatment planning.

LIGHTHALL

In my practice, our multidisciplinary team uses a combination of measures used to evaluate patient outcomes including a subjective physician-graded instrument, objective data, and a patient-reported measure.

At a minimum, all patients are graded using a validated physician-graded instrument. Multiple facial nerve grading instruments have been developed. A systematic review of a the literature evaluating facial nerve grading systems identified the Sunnybrook Facial Grading System as having good intrarater and interrater reliability, and a sensitivity to identifying changes over time, including after therapy.[12] The Sunnybrook Facial Grading System[13] has been evaluated rigorously in the literature and found to have good reliability, allows for static and dynamic assessment, provides a regional evaluation of the face, and incorporates a synkinesis scale. It is my preferred instrument. An emerging physician-graded instrument that has also shown good reliability, an ability to detect changes over time and with intervention, and good correlation with the Sunnybrook Facial Grading System, is the electronic clinician-graded scale to assess facial function, the eFACE.[7,14] The eFACE provides an electronic platform for grading facial function (including on mobile devices), is simple to use, and provides a graphical depiction of function over time and in response to therapy. It may gain widespread use in the future. However, this instrument is not yet part of our routine assessment.

Several validated, easy-to-administer, disease-specific PROMs exist and show good usefulness for the facial paralysis population.[15] We now incorporate a PROM into our assessment battery and prefer the FaCE scale (**Fig. 2**).[2] This scale allows the patient to identify functional deficits and includes questions regarding the impact of their facial paralysis on social interactions. Alterations in these impairments may be followed over time to assess recovery of function or in response to treatment.

Finally, we incorporate standardized photographic views of patients with facial paralysis. We routinely use the 10 views that were proposed as guidelines by Santosa and colleagues[9] to evaluate symmetry in repose as well as to incorporate an assessment of all facial nerve branches to optimize communication between providers. These views allow standardized comparison of outcomes. We also recognize the limitations of photos and now incorporate videography of patients. Ideally, standardized videographic documentation should be obtained with precise patient positioning with the use of standardized facial movements and a smile assay. However,

You may have answered these or similar questions before. Please answer ALL QUESTIONS as best you can.
The following statements are about how you think your face is moving.

(CIRCLE only ONE number)	One side	Both sides	I have no difficulty
When I try to move my face, I find that I have difficulty on	1	2	0

(If you have problems on BOTH sides, answer the questions in the remainder of the survey with regard to the more affected side, or with regard to both sides if they are equally affected.) In the PAST WEEK:

(CIRCLE only ONE number on each line)	Not at all	Only if I concentrate	A little	Almost normally	Normally
1. When I smile, the affected side of my mouth goes up	1	2	3	4	5
2. I can raise my eyebrow on the affected side	1	2	3	4	5
3. When I pucker my lips, the affected side of my mouth moves	1	2	3	4	5

The following are statements about how you might feel because of your FACE OR FACIAL PROBLEM.
Please rate how often each of the following statements applied to you during the PAST WEEK.

(CIRCLE only ONE number on each line)	All of the time	Most of the time	Some of the time	A little of the time	None of the time
4. Parts of my face feel tight, worn out, or uncomfortable	1	2	3	4	5
5. My affected eye feels dry, irritated, or scratchy	1	2	3	4	5
6. When I try to move my face, I feel tension, pain or spasm	1	2	3	4	5
7. I use eye drops or ointment in my affected eye	1	2	3	4	5
8. My affected eye is wet or has tears in it	1	2	3	4	5
9. I act differently around people because of my face or facial problem	1	2	3	4	5
10. People treat me differently because of my face or facial problem	1	2	3	4	5
11. I have problems moving food around in my mouth	1	2	3	4	5
12. I have problems with drooling or keeping food or drink in my mouth or off my chin and clothes	1	2	3	4	5

The following are statements about how you might have felt or been doing in the PAST WEEK
because of your FACE OR FACIAL PROBLEM. Please rate how much you agree with each statement:

(CIRCLE only ONE number on each line)	Strongly agree	Agree	Don't know	Disagree	Strongly disagree
13. My face feels tired or when I try to move my face, I feel tension, pain, or spasm	1	2	3	4	5
14. My appearance has affected my willingness to participate in social activities or to see family or friends	1	2	3	4	5
15. Because of difficulty with the way I eat, I have avoided eating in restaurants or in other people's homes	1	2	3	4	5

Additional comments:

Fig. 2. Facial clinimetric evaluation (FaCE) scale. (From Kahn JB, Gilklich RE, Boyev KP, et al. Validation of a patient-graded instrument for facial nerve paralysis: the FaCE scale. Laryngoscope 2001;111(3):397; with permission.)

this step may be difficult in some practice settings where a dedicated photography/videography suite is not available.

At a minimum, the current assessment battery for patients with facial paralysis should incorporate a physician-graded instrument, a PROM, and photographic/videographic documentation.

Question 2: Are there any techniques that you have migrated away from using and what *have you replaced them with? In which clinical situations would you still use these procedures?*

TOLLEFSON

Over the last 5 to 8 years, I have migrated away from the following 3 techniques: (1) static facial suspension with percutaneous suture suspension of midface, (2) tensor fascia lata facial slings in the setting of radiation treatment, and (3) combination full-thickness skin grafting to the lower eyelid with lower eyelid shortening procedures. I have transitioned from these procedures owing to both dissatisfaction with the results and finding other options to be more effective.

I was disappointed with the duration of effect using percutaneous sutures through the nasolabial fold to suspend the lateral commissure and midface for patients with flaccid facial paralysis.[16] The relapse seen over the first year was consistent. Attempts to thwart relapse using different sutures was ineffective, because the soft tissue pulls through.[17] In response, I began using tensor fascia lata or palmaris longis facial slings to statically position the lateral commissure and create a nasolabial fold. The results were more consistent and predictably long lasting, with the exception being in those patients treated with radiation therapy. Locoregional radiation causes dermal atrophy and sclerosis, which impairs healing and adaptation of even an autologous facial sling material. For these reasons, I now use an orthodromic temporalis tendon transfer in these cases. Although the dynamic effects of the temporalis tendon transfer are attenuated in the radiated field, the static suspension seems to be permanent and effective (**Fig. 3**).

Patients treated with a radical parotidectomy with facial nerve sacrifice and skin resection are prone to refractory lower eyelid retraction and ectropion. This is particularly true in older patients who have also undergone radiation therapy. The resulting combination of cicatricial and paralytic ectropion represents a unique subclass of eyelid malposition.

Theoretically, this conundrum would require procedures that address a lax middle lamella, while addressing cicatricial ectropion and retraction by augmenting the anterior lamella with a skin graft. The first 20 results (Tollefson, unpublished data, 2017) did not show a long-term benefit of using a postauricular full-thickness skin graft to the lower eyelid in these patients. I believe that midface pull on the lower eyelid is the ultimate culprit and, therefore, address this with either a masseteric nerve transfer to a buccal branch or orthodromic temporalis tendon transfer. In the upcoming sections, I further discuss my preference for lower eyelid management using a modified tarsoconjunctival flap.

HADLOCK

I do not really use regional muscle transfer anymore. I do still see patients who have had a masseter muscle transfer elsewhere, but it tends to lead to an unacceptable contour deficit over the mandible. With the temporalis muscle or tendon transfer, the inset is so nuanced that it is less predictable in regard to commissure excursion and resting muscle tension. With optimal results, outcomes can be very good. However, results are not consistently good in my hands and that variability is something that limits its use in my practice. Some groups have extensive experience with this technique and their outcomes are very good, with the average smile excursion being about 4 mm in this patient population.[18,19] When this result is compared with the average excursion obtained from dynamic free tissue transfer, where the average excursion is 7 to 10 mm,[20] most patients

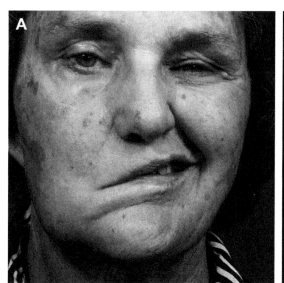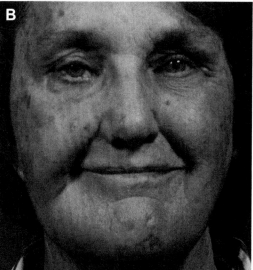

Fig. 3. (*A*) Preoperative photograph of a 60-year-old woman with flaccid (irreversible) facial paralysis. (*B*) One year after orthodromic temporalis tendon transfer. Elevated lateral commissure and lower eyelid supported noted.

in my experience will obtain a better result with free tissue transfer. At my institution, reanimation with free tissue transfer has a very low complication rate in appropriately selected patients and is therefore the treatment of choice.

I also do very few hypoglossal to facial nerve (XII–VII) transfers using the main trunk of the hypoglossal nerve. This is because we now have tools available that provide improved zonal reconstruction than what is achieved with the XII–VII transfer and avoids the donor nerve morbidity. Although modifications of this technique are used, I have not embraced the operation because I have found it difficult for patients to learn to use it and, in my experience, I can obtain better results with other techniques.

LIGHTHALL

I do not use the hypoglossal-to-facial nerve (XII–VII) transfer as a primary procedure or partial hypoglossal transfer. This is primarily due to unacceptable secondary dysfunction owing to donor site deficiencies from hemitongue atrophy, such as dysarthria and dysphagia. Additionally, it is difficult for patients, even with intensive physical therapy, to obtain reliable smile results.[21] This has been mitigated by hemihypoglossal to facial nerve anastomosis as either a primary procedure or as a babysitter procedure before free or regional muscle transfer with acceptable results noted by some authors.[22] However, in my practice, I prefer to use the masseteric to facial nerve transfer when possible. This procedure still requires patients to participate in therapy, but tends to provide stronger and more consistent results. However, at times the reanimated side may develop stronger contractions than the unaffected side (**Fig. 4**). In comparing the hemihypoglossal to facial nerve anastomosis with a masseteric nerve to facial nerve transposition, the latter avoids the donor site morbidity of obtaining a nerve graft and has shown to have improved symmetry with a faster recovery.[23] Currently, there are no clinical situations in which I use the XII–VII procedure.

I also prefer the V–VII nerve transfer or free microneurovascular transfer to muscle transposition in most cases. Clinical situations in which I will incorporate a muscle transposition are in patients with longstanding facial paralysis who have failed a V–VII, are poor candidates for free tissue transfer, or based on patient preference. I no longer transpose temporalis muscle over the arch or use a lengthening temporalis myoplasty owing to donor site morbidity, scarring, and the creation of secondary deformities.[24] When performed, I prefer an orthodromic tendon transfer

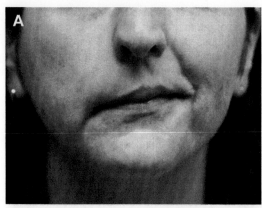

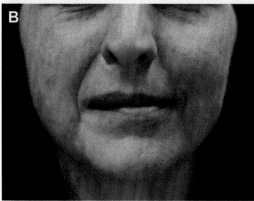

Fig. 4. (*A*) Preoperative photograph of a patient with adenoid cystic carcinoma. (*B*) At 13 months after a masseteric-to-facial nerve transfer and facial rehabilitative therapy.

using either an incision in the melolabial fold or using a transbuccal approach, and may include fascia lata for tendon lengthening.[18,25]

Finally, for treatment of the periocular region, I rarely perform a permanent tarsorrhaphy because it produces an unsightly secondary deformity. I perform a permanent tarsorrhaphy in elderly patients with significant exposure keratopathy or those who have failed other reconstructive options (eg, the posttumor ablative patient who underwent radiation) to allow for immediate corneal protection. Additionally, patients who have combined VIIth and Vth cranial nerve palsies with an insensate cornea may require this procedure. However, aggressive conservative therapy with close follow-up remains the first step in management and can often avoid this procedure. I may perform a tarsorrhaphy for persistent or worsening corneal health, or as an interim measure before being fitted with a fluid-ventilated scleral lens,[26] or while awaiting corneal neurotization from the contralateral supratrochlear nerve.[27]

Question 3: What is the role of nonsurgical treatments and surgical therapies (eg, neurectomy, myectomy) in the treatment of patients with postparesis synkinesis in your practice? What are the limitations of these therapies?

TOLLEFSON

Nonsurgical adjunctive procedures are integral to the comprehensive management of facial paralysis. I will discuss 2 areas: (1) combined neuromuscular retraining/chemodenervation and (2) injectable filler use in deficit perioral and periorbital soft tissue. During recovery from facial paralysis, the hyperdynamic and uncoordinated facial movements can be as frustrating as the facial paralysis. My preference for synkinesis treatment is a team approach involving a neuromuscular retraining specialist and a graduated chemodenervation schedule. Physical therapy traditionally used mirrors and biofeedback to guide a patient in relearning facial movements.[28] Neuromuscular retraining combines a holistic approach to teaching how the synkinetic motions feel and unbundling the imbalances of facial expressions. The specialist then provides a precise plan for botulinum toxin placement to work in accordance with the retraining exercises (**Fig. 5**).

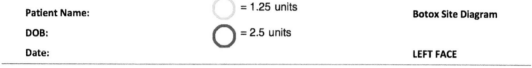

Patient Name: ⭕ = 1.25 units   **Botox Site Diagram**

DOB: ⭕ = 2.5 units

Date: **LEFT FACE**

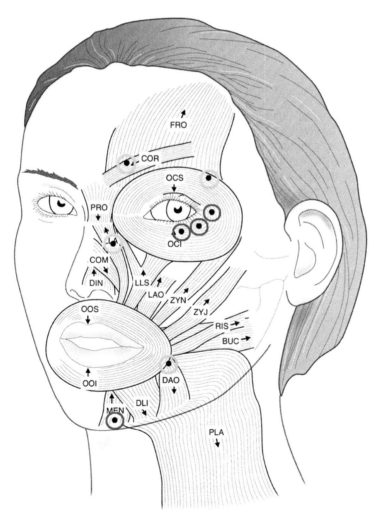

Fig. 5. Chemodenervation planning sheet showing the units of botulinum toxin and sites to be injected. Facial retraining is completed collaboratively to achieve the best results. DAO, depressor anguli oris; DLI, depressor labii inferioris. (*Courtesy of* Jackie Diels, OT, Facial Retraining, LLC, McFarland, WI.)

The major limitation is the lack of availability to trained specialists and lack of insurance coverage, which is partially addressed with the availability of telehealth consultations.[29]

Injectable filler materials provide an office-based, low-risk option to fine tune the volume discrepancies of the lips and, more rarely, the lower eyelid. When reviewing quality-of-life assessments with these patients, they often mention 2 common complaints: difficulty with being understood on the telephone and frustration with eating or drinking in public. I prefer hyaluronic acid fillers and can choose the viscoelastic properties of the available products to match the target goal. Adding volume to the upper and lower lip on the paralyzed side can improve lip apposition, which is so important for consonant pronunciation and drinking (**Fig. 6**). When I am using botulinum toxin on the functional forehead, crow's feet, and lower lip every 3 months, then the filler is placed every 9 months. On the rare occasion that the filler is placed too superficially or seems to be abnormal, hyaluronidase is helpful and effective.

HADLOCK

Chemodenervation of synkinetic muscles is still the gold standard treatment for synkinesis. Before proceeding with neurectomy or myomectomy, patients have to have failed conservative chemodenervation with multiple toxins (eg, Botox and Dysport). Highly selective neurectomies continue to gain traction for the treatment of refractory synkinesis. I do not perform these procedures just because patients do not like getting serial injections because there

is a real risk with highly selective neurectomies to overweaken the muscle of concern. We perform highly selective neurectomies mostly around the periocular region for the treatment of ocular synkinesis performed in a 2-stage procedure with patients awake.[30] We selectively cut 1 branch at a time to provide enough weakening to treat the synkinesis without affecting eye closure. However, if patients are getting good results with serial injections, we continue with that strategy.

We may also perform platysmal denervation by performing either a cervical branch neurectomy or a complete myomectomy of the platysma muscle. The issue with performing cervical neurectomy is that, in some patients, there is a contribution to lower lip bulk, and division of the cervical branch may then create a secondary disfigurement. One of the reasons for that is there are varying contributions of the cervical branch to the lower lip musculature and it is not very predictable. Even with intraoperative stimulation of the cervical branch, it is difficult to predict the outcome owing to the degree of synkinetic movement present and simultaneous coactivation of muscles.

The other thing that is new and emerging is that we are doing a lot of injections to the depressor anguli oris (DAO) muscle. This is probably the single biggest breakthrough in the past 18 months. Dr Labbe[31] in France described cutting out the DAO or weakening it with chemodenervation, and this has been a new topic of discussion at conferences. At our institution, we performed DAO injections with local anesthetic on patients with unilateral facial palsy with DAO synkinesis. We found improved oral commissure excursion and

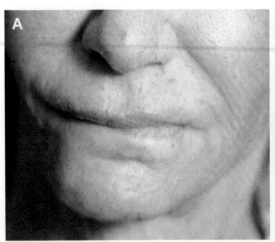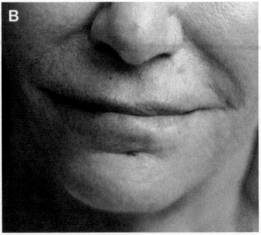

Fig. 6. Patient with lip incompetence, drooling, and dysarthria owing to lower division facial paralysis after extensive mandibular/soft tissue resection reconstructed with fibular free flap. (*A*) Before and (*B*) after injection of 2 mL of hyaluronic acid filler to the right lower lip and commissure and 4 U of botulinum toxin to the contralateral left depressor labii inferioris muscle.

smile symmetry as well as a higher number of naïve observers rating patients as expressing a positive emotion after injection.[32] We have found that about 80% of patients who have good results with local anesthetic injections to the DAO successfully respond to chemodenervation with botulinum toxin and have shown improvement, and not just in adults, but also pediatric patients.[33]

Another newer area of treatment being evaluated in the synkinetic patient is transmucosal chemodenervation of the buccinator muscle for patients who exhibit tightness and synkinesis intraorally and whose oral commissures are drawn straight backward.[34] Contrary to what we have found with the DAO injections, only about 50% of patients who respond to local anesthetic injections into the buccinator when converted to botulinum toxin have an acceptable improvement in their smile without an unacceptable weakening of their lower lip. For these 2 areas (DAO and buccinator muscles), we always perform a trial with a local anesthetic before converting to botulinum toxin. For other areas, based on experience, I know that I can obtain reliable results with chemodenervation of the periocular muscles, contralateral frontalis, and depressor labii inferioris. However, depending on each individual's synkinesis pattern, I cannot assume they are synkinetic in the DAO or the buccinator, and it is not as simple to determine their unique combination of hyperfunction and hypofunction. Therefore, injections of local anesthesia can help to guide treatment.

Finally, physical therapists continue to play an important role in treating the synkinetic patient and optimizing outcomes. Their experience using neuromuscular retraining techniques has become more codified and therapists as a group have gained more experience and have made great strides in terms of preoperative and postoperative manipulation and therapy.

LIGHTHALL

Facial rehabilitation with neuromuscular retraining is essential for the treatment of synkinesis. All new patients undergo 3 months of therapy with a trained facial rehabilitation specialist before initiating any other treatments, because some patients obtain adequate control with therapy alone. Upon reevaluation, if they continue to have troublesome synkinetic movements, then we will then move forward with a trial of chemodenervation to the areas of concern in addition to continuing physical therapy. The majority of patients will obtain good results with this regimen and return every 3 to 4 months for serial injections. This protocol is used for both adults and children who are able to participate in the program. Although most patients will obtain good results with this

protocol, some will have severe or persistent synkinesis that requires surgical therapy.

The most used surgical treatments for synkinesis is platysmal myectomy, which can be done in clinic.[35] For patients with both synkinesis on the affected side and asymmetry owing to persistent weakness, a combination of therapies is typically used to optimize results, including botulinum toxin injections, physical therapy, and deanimation of the contralateral musculature (eg, botulinum toxin or myectomy of the lower lip depressors on the unaffected side).[36]

Although some authors have reported good results with selective neurectomy, this does have a risk of recurrent synkinesis and overweakening the muscle of concern, causing secondary functional deficits such as poor eye closure. The highly selective neurectomy, as described by the Massachusetts Eye and Ear group, has shown good results for refractory synkinesis,[30] but I have limited experience in my practice because the majority of patients do well with serial chemodenervation in combination with an aggressive facial rehabilitation program.

Question 4: When using free muscle transfer for reanimation, what modifications or pearls can you offer to optimize outcomes?

TOLLEFSON

Gracilis free muscle transfer is an effective and relatively consistent method to create perioral facial movement. The nuance is achieving a more natural result that is perceived in the range of normal. This task is difficult, even for the leaders in this field. The technical pearl that I learned from some of these experts is to maintain a fat plane under the dissection in the cheek. This measure can minimize the dermal adhesions to the muscle transfer, which create an unpleasing skin contraction during activation of the smile (**Fig. 7**).

The accurate nasolabial fold creation is imperative, both when inserting a gracilis muscle into the modiolus of the lateral and upper lip, and when inserting an orthodromic temporalis tendon transfer. Knowledge of and mimicry of the native anatomic insertions can be helpful. For example, an insertion that simply duplicates the zygomaticus major muscle creates a lateral pull that is unnatural. Many investigators have written about the Mona Lisa smile, where a small amount of lateral incisor show is seen owing to the vertical vector of the levator labii superioris.[19] Three categories of smile were identified by Rubin in 1974.[37] The most common was the "Mona Lisa" smile (67%), followed by the canine smile (31%), and the "denture" smile (2%).[38] Thus, the category of smile on the patient's functional side should be heeded for the insertions of the

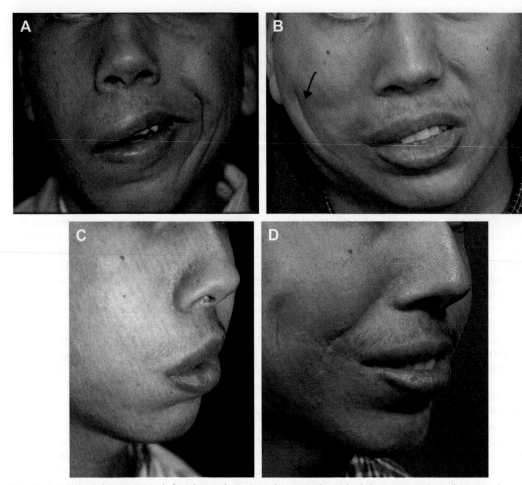

Fig. 7. Patient with congenital facial paralysis (Moebius syndrome). (*A*) Preoperative photograph and (*B*) 6 months after right gracilis muscle transfer innervated by the masseteric nerve, which is demonstrating the abnormal insertions of the gracilis muscle to the right cheek and perioral regions. (*C*) Preoperative oblique view and (*D*) oblique view 9 months after nasolabial fold revision of gracilis muscle insertion.

muscle transfer, often providing movement that is in between the vector of these 2 muscle groups.[39]

HADLOCK

We have made many modifications in our free gracilis technique. We no longer use single innervation cross-facial nerve grafting in patients greater than 30 years old unless they do not have any other neural source. We prefer the masseteric branch of the trigeminal nerve as a single neural source for reanimation, and we have demonstrated excellent excursion of the oral commissure.[20] However, we do many more dually innervated free flaps using both cross-facial nerve grafting and the masseteric branch of the trigeminal nerve. If we use the cross-facial nerve graft with the masseteric branch of the trigeminal nerve, we bring it long and bank it just under the zygomatic arch on the paralyzed side. When we return for the second stage procedure, after we

find the masseteric branch, we can easily identify the end of the cross-facial nerve graft in the adjacent area so that the obturator nerve can have an end-to-end neurorrhaphy for fascicular alignment. At this time, we do not have enough long-term experience with the dually innervated flap to give success rates and quantification of excursion in comparison with flaps innervated with a single neural source.

In general, we are moving toward highly tailored free muscle transfer for reanimation. We are now using almost exclusively the gracilis muscle ipsilateral to the side of paralysis. For years, we were always using different segments of the right gracilis, but were noticing there was more bulkiness when it was transferred to the contralateral face, possibly owing to the region of the muscle that is lying over the zygomatic arch. This problem occurs when the thickest part of muscle in dynamic motion overlies the arch. This issue has not been observed as often with using the ipsilateral muscle in our experience. Further, we have become aggressive about thinning the gracilis and will weigh the muscle intraoperatively with a goal weight of 18 g or less; some flaps have weighed as little as 6 to 10 g with good results. This maneuver decreases the likelihood of excess midface bulk, which creates a secondary disfigurement without increasing the risk of vascular loss or compromising excursion.

With experience, we have been broadening the criteria for candidacy for free tissue transfer. Although younger patients tend to do better with the gracilis free flap, we have obtained excellent smile results with patients in their 70s with limited anesthetic risks. The surgery is now performed with 2 simultaneous surgical teams and, with experience, this procedure now takes about 4 to 5 hours of total operating time.

Free tissue transfer for reanimation has classically been reserved for patients with flaccid facial paralysis. However, we have been performing this procedure for quite a long time in patients with non-flaccid facial paralysis or "frozen faces" with good outcomes.[40]

There are several other modifications of the gracilis flap. We are now insetting the muscle with 2 vectors so that we are also treating the lip elevators. In the frozen face, we are exenterating the platysma at the same time as the gracilis free flap. We are also experimenting with a concurrent DAO to depressor labii inferioris pedicled muscle transfer. This procedure involves taking the DAO off of the modiolus and transferring it to the midline of the lower lip such that, when it activates, it replaces the motion of the depressor labii inferioris. We are in the infancy of this operation with only a few cases performed so far. Greater numbers are needed to evaluate clinical outcomes.

I suspect that as we gain additional experience and comfort with highly tailored free flaps, the criteria will be further expanded to optimize results for patients with facial paralysis.

LIGHTHALL

My facial nerve practice continues to undergo modifications with increasing experience and continued discussions with colleagues. Several pearls that were imprinted on me by experts with many years of experience can help to achieve reliable results. First, patient selection is critical, particularly when first establishing a facial nerve practice. Although a spontaneous smile is the goal, patients still require physical therapy to optimize results. We will have all patients with a planned reanimation procedure undergo a prehabilitation program where they work with a facial

therapist before surgery for counseling, to learn postoperative facial exercises, and to provide patients with videos of exercises they will perform. They will then work with the therapist after surgery to maximize results.

In general, the trend was to use a sural cross-facial nerve graft with delayed second stage free tissue transfer. We then saw the emergence of single-staged flaps innervated by the masseteric nerve with some reports of improved excursion and strength, with concerns for possible decreased spontaneity.[41] Now, we prefer the single-staged dually innervated flaps using both a sural cross-facial nerve graft in conjunction with the masseteric nerve, which has been shown to have good outcomes with relation to the degree of oral commissure excursion, strength of the flap, and provides spontaneity of the smile.[20,42,43] Currently, the ideal flap innervation is yet to be determined and larger studies with long-term results comparing innervation are necessary.

With free tissue transfer, there is a tendency is to leave a greater amount of muscle to provide contractile force or for fear that aggressive thinning may compromise the vascular supply and lead to flap loss. This measure may lead to a secondary deformity duet of excess muscle bulk in the midface and over the arch. Although we do not yet know the ideal weight or length of flap to harvest, sequential thinning of the flap is safe and intraoperative muscle stimulation will help to confirm adequate muscle contraction. Collecting intraoperative details on muscle length at rest and during stimulation, width of muscle, and muscle weight are key to assist in continuing to find the perfect balance between aesthetics and function.

Finally, performing other procedures at the same as a free gracilis transfer such as a mini temporalis transfer to lower eyelid, adding a slip of fascia lata to nasal base or to support the lower eyelid, or treating contralateral lower lip depressors may optimize results based on patient needs.

Question 5: What do you see as the future of treatment for patients with facial paralysis and what are key areas where research should focus?

TOLLEFSON

The schedule for an upcoming International Facial Nerve Society Symposium includes a panel on technology and future applications, which illustrate the diverse work in facial paralysis research. Two of these areas are bioengineering devices and advances in neurografts. I began work on using artificial muscle to restore blink through an eyelid sling mechanism in 2007 (**Fig. 8**).[44] After determining the force and vector requirements,

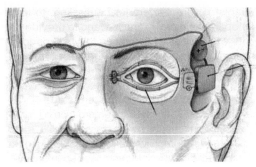

Fig. 8. Illustration of eyelid sling prototype, which is powered by an electroactive polymer artificial muscle implanted into the temporal fossa. (*From* Senders C, Tollefson T, Curtiss S, et al. Force requirements for artificial muscle to create an eyelid blink with eyelid sling. Arch Facial Plast Surg 2010;12(1):31; with permission.)

we implanted electroactive polymer artificial muscle devices into a rodent model and achieved function for months in vivo. The limitation that has stalled the work at this point is the excessive size of polymer device needed to create eyelid closure in the cadaver model. Several groups have continued to devise methods to create eyelid closure using a sling device, and others are concentrating on an external sling that blinks the eye.[45] All of these ideas require synchronization with the functional eye, which have been postulated using electromyographic signal or infrared detectors on glasses.[46]

In the treatment of acute facial paralysis, promising results have been shown with facial pacing, a treatment with a closed-loop neuroprosthetic device that is being developed at Massachusetts Eye and Ear Infirmary.[46,47] A controversial area exists in Functional Electrical Stimulation devices, which give small, brief electrical pulses to paralyzed muscles. These devices have gained attention in patients with spinal cord injuries, and some investigators are reporting its use in facial paralysis.[48]

Repairing facial nerve defects with nerve guide conduits is the other promising research area. For peripheral nerve defects, there are a variety of nerve guide conduits available that can be used off the shelf, but these are yet to become common practice in facial paralysis. Three-dimensional printed nerve bioconduits are an exciting advance in the peripheral nerve arena, which may translate to facial paralysis.[49] There is ongoing research into the use of a peptide amphiphile nanofiber conduit that may guide neural growth through the nanostructure.[50] The potential benefits of a successful nerve conduit include decreasing donor site morbidity and surgical time.

HADLOCK

Currently, the trend is for early reinnervation. We no longer feel it is acceptable that a patient with flaccid paralysis 6 months after a skull base surgery to wait the additional 6 months to provide reinnervation to the native musculature. The Hopkins group has shown this nicely and our results are in complete alignment.[51] Once you know there will be unacceptable recovery, you should reinnervate at the earliest point. In cases where there is a potential for recovery, this is a hard stop and we will delay innervation to allow maximal spontaneous recovery.

The future of facial reanimation is going to heavily lie in the realm of neural prosthesis work. We are going to have a system whereby movement detection on the good side will stimulate and trigger movement on the paralyzed side. In other words, there will be a neural prosthetic device whereby movement on the paralyzed side will be driven by normal movement on the unaffected side in near real time.[46,47,52]

The second thing we hope to see is the development of targeted suicide substances that will kill inappropriately innervated muscle. So, for example, if we can inject the platysma with a permanent Botox, we can provide long-lasting results.

The other area that we see emerging in the long term is that we are going to get better at molecular manipulation of actual facial nerve regeneration. We will be able to help direct the fibers to regenerate back to their original target and the way we are going to do that is to better understand the subnuclei of the facial motor nucleus. If we look at the neural fingerprint of what the nerve is expressing in the group that is the frontalis muscle innervators, we believe that that profile is different than the fingerprint of the one to the orbicularis oculi or the midface branches. We are trying to develop those profiles so that we can exploit them to achieve more precise directionality of regenerating fibers.[53,54]

Other waves of the future include attempting to quantitate the personal and societal value of facial reanimation procedures. This process includes examining the impact of facial paralysis on quality of life, people's willingness to pay for treatment, and identifying the health utility of interventions for facial paralysis.[55–58] Understanding these factors will help us to stratify surgical and medical priorities for patients with facial paralysis.

We are now also using something called a PROSE lens (Prosthetic Replacement of the Ocular Surface Ecosystem) for the prevention and treatment of exposure keratopathy.[59,60] This contact lens creates the correct microclimate for an inadequately protected cornea and may minimize the need for disfiguring procedures to provide corneal protection. In the future, I expect we will see modifications of the PROSE lens with the possibility of a permanent implant to provide sustained corneal protection. There will also likely be advances in neoneurotization of the cornea in patients with combined facial and trigeminal nerve palsies. Already people are neurotizing the cornea with a sural nerve cable graft from the contralateral supratrochlear, and this procedure is likely to become a surgical technique that will find new adopters.[27]

Finally, I believe we will be moving toward data registries and the development of centers of excellence with a minimum level of cases necessary to maintain this designation. We will likely be required to anonymously or semianonymously provide data in terms of free tissue excursion, complication rates, and PROMs to ensure high-quality care for patients with facial paralysis.

LIGHTHALL

Research and future treatment options for patients with facial paralysis will likely be aimed at improving recovery after injury and minimizing aberrant regeneration during axonal regrowth to prevent synkinesis. A body of research exists that looks at the use of neurotrophic factors and stem cells to promote faster and more complete nerve recovery with less development of aberrant regenerative pathways.[61–63] The ultimate goal would be to either inject, implant, or ingest factors that will optimize and support a healthy microenvironment for targeted axonal growth. At this time, most studies are still in the animal model phase, but we hope to see clinical studies in the near future.

Management of the paralyzed eye remains suboptimal despite our best available treatments. Attempts at restoring eye closure and blink by using contralateral input to provide symmetry and function using either an external or eventually an implantable device is another promising area of research that should be further developed.[46,52] Several of these studies use either an external device, whereas others are evaluating the use of a fully implantable model that will record input from the unaffected side and transmit the data to the paralyzed side to provide a stimulus for a coordinated blink. Other studies have evaluated the use of artificial muscle implantation in addition to a stimulator to provide eye closure.[64]

Finally, as mentioned, for patients with significant exposure keratopathy or with a combined trigeminal and facial insult in which the cornea is insensate in addition to the presence of lagophthalmos and a decreased blink, scleral contact lenses may be fitted to improve the microenvironment of the corneal surface.[26] These lenses are currently available but not widely used because they require specialized fitting and staff, are expensive, and there is poor awareness of their availability.

Question 6: What is the single most important advancement in technique for treatment of facial paralysis that you have adopted in the past 5 years? How else has your facial reanimation practice evolved over the past 5 years?

TOLLEFSON

My experience with managing eyelid function in facial paralysis has benefited greatly from referrals from a vigorous head and neck cancer surgical team. Around a decade ago, I noted that a traditional lateral tarsal strip canthoplasty and gold weight placement were not sufficient for many patients after major oncologic resections. Cornea protection is paramount. Patients often complain of the paradoxic dry eye discomfort along with simultaneous epiphora. In the past 5 years, I have advocated for protective gas-permeable scleral contact lens[26] and added the mini-Hughes tarsoconjunctival flap to my eyelid treatment paradigm.[21]

Many of these referred patients are more than 60 years old, had facial nerve resection with or without cable nerve grafting, free tissue transfers for temporal or midface soft tissue reconstruction, and underwent postoperative radiation therapy. These factors contributed to the very difficult lower eyelid retraction and ectropion, which could be categorized as senile, paralytic, and cicatricial. Each of these types have traditional treatments, including midface lifting, lateral and medial canthoplasty or lower lid shortening, or lower eyelid skin grafting, respectively. Often a lateral tarsorrhaphy procedure was needed when the other techniques failed with this patient population.

The drawback of the permanent tarsorrhaphy is 2-fold: a poor aesthetic result of a partially closed eyelid and peripheral visual field deficit from the narrowed aperture (**Fig. 9**). In the last 3 years, I have adopted a technique described by Sufyan and colleagues,[65] the mini-Hughes or tarsoconjunctival flap along with a tarsal strip canthoplasty. This technique is reversible, adjustable (a larger flap provides more protection), and, most important, protects the cornea on upward gaze (**Fig. 10**). Quality of life was seen to improve with less epiphora, dry eye pain, and need for eye lubrication. As a supportive anecdote, a patient who competes in masters' competitive tennis described improvement in protection from the wind while on the court.

The tarsoconjunctival flap is traditionally a 2-stage procedure for lower eyelid defects

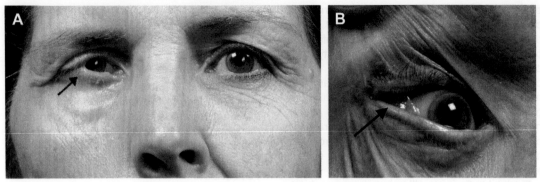

Fig. 9. (*A*) Patient with flaccid, permanent facial paralysis after acoustic neuroma resection with a permanent tarsorrhaphy (*arrow*). Note the poor aesthetic appearance of the tarsorrhaphy compared with a similar patient treated with a (*B*) tarsoconjunctival flap/tarsal strip canthoplasty (*arrow*).

that is divided after several weeks to open the eyelids. In this case, the small flap is left intact. The upper eyelid tarsus and conjunctiva are incised with superiorly based flap that is inset into the lateral lower eyelid gray line. When possible, I use a lateral retinacular suspension at the time of the flap inset to prevent further scarring of the lateral canthal apparatus.[66]

Otherwise, my practice has evolved to include the nuances of combining a simultaneous masseteric nerve and cross-face facial nerve grafting to the buccal and zygomatic branches, respectively.[67] The potential benefit is that the more powerful masseteric nerve can generate a smile, while the eyelid blink would be involuntarily generated from the cross-face innervation (**Fig. 11**). As these techniques and others are evolving, chemodenervation

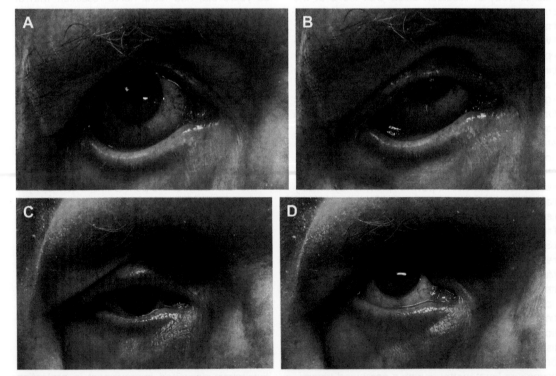

Fig. 10. Patient with flaccid facial paralysis (*A*) before with eyelid open and (*B*) eyelid closed (severe lagophthalmos). (*C*) Paralytic ectropion was treated with a right eyelid mini-Hughes tarsoconjunctival flap performed with a tarsal strip canthoplasty shown 6 months postoperatively. (*D*) Both techniques protect the cornea when the patient looks upward.

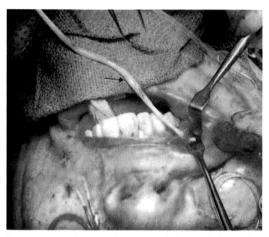

Fig. 11. Cross-face sural nerve graft (*arrow*) shown being passed under upper lip from a functional left zygomatic branch to the paralyzed side.

with botulinum toxin and facial retraining continue to be essential in addressing synkinesis and hyperdynamic function after nerve grafting.

HADLOCK

Use of the masseteric nerve for reanimation both directly with a V–VII transfer and as a single or more often dual innervation source for free muscle transfer. The masseteric to facial nerve (V–VII) transfer came into vogue about 4 to 5 years ago. We began to use it as a single modality for reanimation on a regular basis in all patients, including both the flaccid face and the frozen face. We had excellent results in the flaccid face, but discovered that we had less reliable results in the frozen face. Based on the minimal gain in this population, I think the operation is only useful in the flaccid stage. We also use the V–VII transfer at the time of resection for the radical parotidectomy patient, which is new. If they obtain good results with this technique, then a delayed free tissue transfer may not be necessary. Finally, as noted, we have obtained better oral commissure excursion with free tissue transfer when the masseteric nerve is use alone to innervate a free gracilis transfer. We recently have been using it for dual innervation of the gracilis flaps, although longer term results are necessary to assess outcomes.

The Massachusetts Eye and Ear Infirmary practice continues to evolve to more customized reanimation, including the highly tailored free flaps, the increasing use of highly selective neurectomies, and the development of micromimetic pedicled muscle transfer like the DAO.

However, our hope and goal is that we effectively put ourselves out of business by never wasting the native musculature by providing early reinnervation and eventual neural regeneration to all patients in the future.

LIGHTHALL

Incorporating the masseteric nerve for direct facial nerve coaptation (V–VII transfer) in patients with intact facial musculature or as a neural source for free tissue transfer for patients who have longstanding paralysis with muscle atrophy into my reanimation practice has been the most important advancement I have adopted. The relative ease of dissection[51] intraoperatively, availability as a single-stage procedure for free tissue transfer, strong axonal input leading to excellent results in oral commissure excursion, and avoidance of multiple neural coaptations has made this a popular neural source. Concerns regarding spontaneity of smile produces may be decreased by using the masseteric nerve in conjunction with a cross-facial nerve graft.[68,69]

My facial nerve practice continues to evolve. In the past year, we have created a multidisciplinary facial nerve disorders center that allows for coordinated care, availability of multiple facial rehabilitation specialists, consistency in obtaining clinical outcomes data, and advanced expertise in multiple subspecialties, allowing for holistic patient care. Incorporating a PROM as discussed allows for an assessment of the meaningfulness of the interventions we provide. I suspect the future of treatment for patients with facial paralysis will move toward multidisciplinary centers. Additional multiinstitutional, long-term data on clinical outcomes and changes on patients' quality of life will be instrumental in determining the optimal facial reanimation paradigm.

REFERENCES

1. Ishii LE, Godoy A, Encarnacion CO, et al. What faces reveal: impaired affect display in facial paralysis. Laryngoscope 2011;121(6):1138–43.
2. Kahn JB, Gliklich RE, Boyev KP, et al. Validation of a patient-graded instrument for facial nerve paralysis: the FaCE scale. Laryngoscope 2001;111(3):387–98.
3. Stewart MG, Witsell DL, Smith TL, et al. Development and validation of the nasal obstruction symptom evaluation (NOSE) scale. Otolaryngol Head Neck Surg 2004;130(2):157–63.
4. Hadlock T. Standard outcome measures in facial paralysis: getting on the same page. JAMA Facial Plast Surg 2016;18(2):85–6.
5. Bhama P, Gliklich RE, Weinberg JS, et al. Optimizing total facial nerve patient management for effective clinical outcomes research. JAMA Facial Plast Surg 2014;16(1):9–14.

6. Banks CA, Bhama PK, Park J, et al. Clinician-graded electronic facial paralysis assessment: the eFACE. Plast Reconstr Surg 2015;136(2):223e–30e.

7. Banks CA, Jowett N, Hadlock CR, et al. Weighting of facial grading variables to disfigurement in facial palsy. JAMA Facial Plast Surg 2016;18(4):292–8.

8. Banks CA, Jowett N, Hadlock TA. Test-retest reliability and agreement between in-person and video assessment of facial mimetic function using the eFACE facial grading system. JAMA Facial Plast Surg 2017;19(3):206–11.

9. Santosa KB, Fattah A, Gavilan J, et al. Photographic standards for patients with facial palsy and recommendations by members of the Sir Charles Bell Society. JAMA Facial Plast Surg 2017;19(4):275–81.

10. Hadlock TA, Malo JS, Cheney ML, et al. Free gracilis transfer for smile in children: the Massachusetts eye and ear infirmary experience in excursion and quality-of-life changes. Arch Facial Plast Surg 2011;13(3):190–4.

11. Vrabec JT, Backous DD, Djalilian HR, et al. Facial nerve grading system 2.0. Otolaryngol Head Neck Surg 2009;140(4):445–50.

12. Fattah AY, Gurusinghe AD, Gavilan J, et al. Facial nerve grading instruments: systematic review of the literature and suggestion for uniformity. Plast Reconstr Surg 2015;135(2):569–79.

13. Ross BG, Fradet G, Nedzelski JM. Development of a sensitive clinical facial grading system. Otolaryngol Head Neck Surg 1996;114(3):380–6.

14. Gaudin RA, Robinson M, Banks CA, et al. Emerging vs time-tested methods of facial grading among patients with facial paralysis. JAMA Facial Plast Surg 2016;18(4):251–7.

15. Ho AL, Scott AM, Klassen AF, et al. Measuring quality of life and patient satisfaction in facial paralysis patients: a systematic review of patient-reported outcome measures. Plast Reconstr Surg 2012;130(1):91–9.

16. Tate JR, Tollefson TT. Advances in facial reanimation. Curr Opin Otolaryngol Head Neck Surg 2006;14(4):242–8.

17. Humphrey CD, McIff TE, Sykes KJ, et al. Suture biomechanics and static facial suspension. Arch Facial Plast Surg 2007;9(3):188–93.

18. Boahene KD, Farrag TY, Ishii L, et al. Minimally invasive temporalis tendon transposition. Arch Facial Plast Surg 2011;13(1):8–13.

19. Byrne PJ, Kim M, Boahene K, et al. Temporalis tendon transfer as part of a comprehensive approach to facial reanimation. Arch Facial Plast Surg 2007;9(4):234–41.

20. Bhama PK, Weinberg JS, Lindsay RW, et al. Objective outcomes analysis following microvascular gracilis transfer for facial reanimation: a review of 10 years' experience. JAMA Facial Plast Surg 2014;16(2):85–92.

21. Harris BN, Tollefson TT. Facial reanimation: evolving from static procedures to free tissue transfer in head and neck surgery. Curr Opin Otolaryngol Head Neck Surg 2015;23(5):399–406.

22. Terzis JK, Tzafetta K. "Babysitter" procedure with concomitant muscle transfer in facial paralysis. Plast Reconstr Surg 2009;124(4):1142–56.

23. Hontanilla B, Marre D. Comparison of hemihypoglossal nerve versus masseteric nerve transpositions in the rehabilitation of short-term facial paralysis using the Facial Clima evaluating system. Plast Reconstr Surg 2012;130(5):662e–72e.

24. Moubayed SP, Labbe D, Rahal A. Lengthening temporalis myoplasty for facial paralysis reanimation: an objective analysis of each surgical step. JAMA Facial Plast Surg 2015;17(3):179–82.

25. Owusu Boahene KD. Temporalis muscle tendon unit transfer for smile restoration after facial paralysis. Facial Plast Surg Clin North Am 2016;24(1):37–45.

26. Weyns M, Koppen C, Tassignon MJ. Scleral contact lenses as an alternative to tarsorrhaphy for the long-term management of combined exposure and neurotrophic keratopathy. Cornea 2013;32(3):359–61.

27. Bains RD, Elbaz U, Zuker RM, et al. Corneal neurotization from the supratrochlear nerve with sural nerve grafts: a minimally invasive approach. Plast Reconstr Surg 2015;135(2):397e–400e.

28. Wernick Robinson M, Baiungo J, Hohman M, et al. Facial rehabilitation. Oper Tech Otolaryngol Head Neck Surg 2012;23(4):288–96.

29. Available at: www.Facialretraining.org. Accessed May 17, 2017.

30. Hohman MH, Lee LN, Hadlock TA. Two-step highly selective neurectomy for refractory periocular synkinesis. Laryngoscope 2013;123(6):1385–8.

31. Labbe D, Benichou L, Iodice A, et al. Depressor anguli oris sign (DAO) in facial paresis. How to search it and release the smile (technical note). Ann Chir Plast Esthet 2012;57(3):281–5 [in French].

32. Jowett N, Malka R, Hadlock TA. Effect of weakening of ipsilateral depressor anguli oris on smile symmetry in postparalysis facial palsy. JAMA Facial Plast Surg 2017;19(1):29–33.

33. Haykal S, Arad E, Bagher S, et al. The role of botulinum toxin a in the establishment of symmetry in pediatric paralysis of the lower lip. JAMA Facial Plast Surg 2015;17(3):174–8.

34. Wei LA, Diels J, Lucarelli MJ. Treating buccinator with botulinum toxin in patients with facial synkinesis: a previously overlooked target. Ophthal Plast Reconstr Surg 2016;32(2):138–41.

35. Henstrom DK, Malo JS, Cheney ML, et al. Platysmectomy: an effective intervention for facial synkinesis and hypertonicity. Arch Facial Plast Surg 2011;13(4):239–43.

36. Chen CK, Tang YB. Myectomy and botulinum toxin for paralysis of the marginal mandibular branch of

the facial nerve: a series of 76 cases. Plast Reconstr Surg 2007;120(7):1859–64.

37. Rubin LR. The anatomy of a smile: its importance in the treatment of facial paralysis. Plast Reconstr Surg 1974;53(4):384–7.

38. Rubin LR. The anatomy of the nasolabial fold: the keystone of the smiling mechanism. Plast Reconstr Surg 1999;103(2):687–91 [discussion: 692–4].

39. Sharma PR, Zuker RM, Borschel GH. Gracilis free muscle transfer in the treatment of pediatric facial paralysis. Facial Plast Surg 2016;32(2):199–208.

40. Lindsay RW, Bhama P, Weinberg J, et al. The success of free gracilis muscle transfer to restore smile in patients with nonflaccid facial paralysis. Ann Plast Surg 2014;73(2):177–82.

41. Hontanilla B, Marre D, Cabello A. Facial reanimation with gracilis muscle transfer neurotized to cross-facial nerve graft versus masseteric nerve: a comparative study using the FACIAL CLIMA evaluating system. Plast Reconstr Surg 2013;131(6):1241–52.

42. Biglioli F, Colombo V, Tarabbia F, et al. Double innervation in free-flap surgery for long-standing facial paralysis. J Plast Reconstr Aesthet Surg 2012; 65(10):1343–9.

43. Garcia RM, Hadlock TA, Klebuc MJ, et al. Contemporary solutions for the treatment of facial nerve paralysis. Plast Reconstr Surg 2015;135(6):1025e–46e.

44. Senders CW, Tollefson TT, Curtiss S, et al. Force requirements for artificial muscle to create an eyelid blink with eyelid sling. Arch Facial Plast Surg 2010; 12(1):30–6.

45. Kozaki Y, Suzuki K. A facial wearable robot with eyelid gating mechanism for supporting eye blink. 2016 International Symposium on Micro-NanoMechatronics and Human Science (MHS), Nagoya, 2016. p. 1–5.

46. Frigerio A, Hadlock TA, Murray EH, et al. Infrared-based blink-detecting glasses for facial pacing: toward a bionic blink. JAMA Facial Plast Surg 2014; 16(3):211–8.

47. Frigerio A, Heaton JT, Cavallari P, et al. Electrical stimulation of eye blink in individuals with acute facial palsy: progress toward a bionic blink. Plast Reconstr Surg 2015;136(4):515e–23e.

48. Raslan A, Volk GF, Moller M, et al. High variability of facial muscle innervation by facial nerve branches: a prospective electrostimulation study. Laryngoscope 2017;127(6):1288–95.

49. Hu Y, Wu Y, Gou Z, et al. 3D-engineering of cellularized conduits for peripheral nerve regeneration. Sci Rep 2016;6:32184.

50. Li A, Hokugo A, Yalom A, et al. A bioengineered peripheral nerve construct using aligned peptide amphiphile nanofibers. Biomaterials 2014;35(31):8780–90.

51. Albathi M, Oyer S, Ishii LE, et al. Early nerve grafting for facial paralysis after cerebellopontine angle tumor resection with preserved facial nerve continuity. JAMA Facial Plast Surg 2016;18(1):54–60.

52. Hasmat S, Lovell NH, Suaning GJ, et al. Restoration of eye closure in facial paralysis using implantable electromagnetic actuator. J Plast Reconstr Aesthet Surg 2016;69(11):1521–5.

53. Choi D, Raisman G. Somatotopic organization of the facial nucleus is disrupted after lesioning and regeneration of the facial nerve: the histological representation of synkinesis. Neurosurgery 2002;50(2): 355–62 [discussion: 362–3].

54. Choi D, Raisman G. Disorganization of the facial nucleus after nerve lesioning and regeneration in the rat: effects of transplanting candidate reparative cells to the site of injury. Neurosurgery 2005;56(5): 1093–100 [discussion: 1093–100].

55. Ishii L, Dey J, Boahene KD, et al. The social distraction of facial paralysis: objective measurement of social attention using eye-tracking. Laryngoscope 2016;126(2):334–9.

56. Ishii L, Godoy A, Encarnacion CO, et al. Not just another face in the crowd: society's perceptions of facial paralysis. Laryngoscope 2012;122(3):533–8.

57. Nellis JC, Ishii M, Byrne PJ, et al. Association among facial paralysis, depression, and quality of life in facial plastic surgery patients. JAMA Facial Plast Surg 2017;19(3):190–6.

58. Su P, Ishii LE, Joseph A, et al. Societal value of surgery for facial reanimation. JAMA Facial Plast Surg 2017;19(2):139–46.

59. Gire A, Kwok A, Marx DP. PROSE treatment for lagophthalmos and exposure keratopathy. Ophthal Plast Reconstr Surg 2013;29(2):e38–40.

60. Chahal JS, Heur M, Chiu GB. Prosthetic replacement of the ocular surface ecosystem scleral lens therapy for exposure keratopathy. Eye Contact Lens 2017;43(4):240–4.

61. Grosheva M, Nohroudi K, Schwarz A, et al. Comparison of trophic factors' expression between paralyzed and recovering muscles after facial nerve injury. A quantitative analysis in time course. Exp Neurol 2016;279:137–48.

62. Abbas OL, Borman H, Uysal CA, et al. Adipose-derived stem cells enhance axonal regeneration through cross-facial nerve grafting in a rat model of facial paralysis. Plast Reconstr Surg 2016;138(2):387–96.

63. Wang TV, Delaney S, Pepper JP. Current state of stem cell-mediated therapies for facial nerve injury. Curr Opin Otolaryngol Head Neck Surg 2016;24(4):285–93.

64. Ledgerwood LG, Tinling S, Senders C, et al. Artificial muscle for reanimation of the paralyzed face: durability and biocompatibility in a gerbil model. Arch Facial Plast Surg 2012;14(6):413–8.

65. Sufyan AS, Lee HB, Shah H, et al. Single-stage repair of paralytic ectropion using a novel modification of the tarsoconjunctival flap. JAMA Facial Plast Surg 2014;16(2):151–2.

66. Fagien S. Algorithm for canthoplasty: the lateral retinacular suspension: a simplified suture canthopexy.

Plast Reconstr Surg 1999;103(7):2042–53 [discussion: 2054–8].

67. Biglioli F, Bayoudh W, Colombo V, et al. Double innervation (facial/masseter) on the gracilis flap, in the middle face reanimation in the management of facial paralysis: a new concept. Ann Chir Plast Esthet 2013;58(2):89–95 [in French].

68. Biglioli F, Colombo V, Rabbiosi D, et al. Masseteric-facial nerve neurorrhaphy: results of a case series. J Neurosurg 2017;126(1):312–8.

69. Snyder-Warwick AK, Fattah AY, Zive L, et al. The degree of facial movement following microvascular muscle transfer in pediatric facial reanimation depends on donor motor nerve axonal density. Plast Reconstr Surg 2015;135(2):370e–81e.

Management of the Prominent Ear

Andres Gantous, MD, FRCS(C)[a],*, Abel-Jan Tasman, MD[b], Jose Carlos Neves, MD[c,d]

KEYWORDS

- Otoplasty • Incisionless otoplasty • Ear setback surgery • Prominent ears • Ear cosmetic surgery
- Ear surgery

KEY POINTS

- The role of nonsurgical management of the prominent ear is discussed by presenting some traditional and current concepts available as well as investigational future trends.
- Current concepts in the management of prominent ears are presented from North American and European perspectives.
- The role of cartilage-cutting and cartilage-sparing otoplasty is discussed as well as management options for the prominent ear lobe.
- Postoperative management of patients undergoing different types of otoplasty is discussed.

 Video content accompanies this article at http://www.facialplastic.theclinics.com.

Panel discussion

1. What is the role for nonsurgical management of the prominent ear?

2. What are the advantages and disadvantages of cartilage-sparing techniques compared with cartilage-cutting techniques when modifying or recreating the antihelical fold?

3. What is your preferred surgical technique when performing otoplasty? What are the indications and contraindications for this technique in your hands? If you do not perform your usual technique, what other techniques do you perform?

4. How do you deal with the prominent ear lobe?

5. How do you manage your otoplasty patients postoperatively?

6. What are the sociocultural and technical considerations in performing otoplasty in nonwhite patients?

7. How have your techniques in this area changed over the past 5 years?

Disclosure Statement: The authors have nothing to disclose.
[a] Department of Otolaryngology–Head and Neck Surgery, Division of Facial Plastic and Reconstructive Surgery, University of Toronto, 30 The Queensway SSW 230, Toronto, Ontario M6R 1B5, Canada; [b] Rhinology, Facial Plastic Surgery, ENT-Department, Cantonal Hospital St. Gallen, Hals-Nasen-Ohrenklinik, Rorschacher Strasse 95, St Gallen CH-9007, Switzerland; [c] My Face, Clinica da Face, Avenida Miguel Bombarda # 36, 8 D, Saldanha, Lisboa 1050-165, Portugal; [d] My Face, Clinica da Face, Coimbra, Portugal
* Corresponding author.
E-mail address: drgantous@torontofacialplastic.com

Facial Plast Surg Clin N Am 26 (2018) 181–192
https://doi.org/10.1016/j.fsc.2017.12.010

Question 1: What is the role for nonsurgical management of the prominent ear?

GANTOUS

Prominauris, or prominent ears, is the most common congenital deformity of the head and neck area. It is estimated that its incidence is 5% in the white population as an autosomal dominant trait, but the incidence of auricular deformities has been estimated to be as high as 47% of all births.[1,2] A common but erroneous belief held by many health practitioners is that a majority of ear deformities detected in newborns correct themselves with time. In truth, only a third of these deformities self-correct.[3] Another misconception is that these minor cosmetic defects cause minimal psychological effects or problems of adjustment. MacGregor[4] has shown that in deviations that provoked laughter or were objects of ridicule or derogatory nicknames, the psychological impact was marked.

It has been found that the auricular cartilage has unusual plasticity during the first few weeks of life. The high levels of circulating estrogen peak at day 3, returning to a baseline level by the sixth week of life. It is thought that hyaluronic acid is elevated by the high estrogen levels and is responsible for the increased plasticity and malleability of the newborn cartilage.[2] The nonsurgical correction of auricular deformities using a variety of splinting techniques was first described in the 1980s in several publications from Japan.[2,5,6] Excellent results have been reported when the ear molding is carried out within the first 6 weeks of life for a variety of auricular deformities of varying severity. Furthermore, Tan and colleagues[7] have shown a 4% rate of residual deformity compared with a 10% to 24% rate with surgery.

An effort should be made to educate pediatricians, obstetricians, midwives, and nurses to identify these deformities early on before the window for nonsurgical intervention closes. This may reduce the need for future surgical correction in these children.[8]

TASMAN

Depending on the semantic definition of "nonsurgical," a facial plastic surgeon may only speculate on the potential role of techniques that ideally complement the classical surgical armamentarium. Understanding "nonsurgical" in a broad sense as not based on the cutting of tissues, bracing of the pinna in the first weeks of life, laser-assisted heat-induced reshaping of auricular cartilage, and incisionless suture-based techniques deserves mentioning.

Taking advantage of a window of opportunity in which the future shape of the auricle can be changed by molding the cartilage was initially described in the 1980s. Early reports of successful corrections by taping the auricle were followed by the use of foam and, later, the development of a molding system.[3] A later report suggested reducing the duration of the molding period to as short as 2 weeks, if the treatment can be started within the first days postnatum.[9] This author, having no personal experience with the technique, speculates that the role of this truly nonsurgical treatment may grow in the future. Another treatment that may be considered nonsurgical has been named laser-assisted cartilage reshaping. The treatment principle is based on weakening the cartilage by heating it to 65°C to 75°C and then bringing it into a desired shape with a silastic elastomer.[10] Thermal energy is applied transcutaneously to the cartilage with lasers of different wavelengths, of which the 1540-nm Er:glass laser produced what the investigators called favorable results with little thermal damage to the auricular skin and no need for local anesthesia. The incidence of damage to the skin, reported to be higher with the 1064-nm Nd:YAG laser,[11] the limited availability of the preferred Er:glass laser, and the need to splint the auricle for several weeks may limit the acceptance of this technique in the facial plastic surgery community. Suture-based incisionless otoplasty techniques, initially described by Fritsch[12] in the early 1990s, continue to be a fascinating alternative to open surgical approaches, with convincing esthetic long-term results and acceptable complication and revision rates.[13] Incisionless techniques are appealing and the published results are convincing. This author, having no personal experience with this nonsurgical technique either, still prefers the versatility of a surgical approach, for rigid cartilage in particular.

Question 2: What are the advantages and disadvantages of cartilage-sparing techniques compared with cartilage-cutting techniques when modifying or recreating the antihelical fold?

GANTOUS

This is a question that has been brought up, discussed, and been a source of animosity between the camps promoting one over the other.

Mustarde[14] first described the use of permanent sutures to recreate the antihelical fold and it is probably the most widely taught and used cartilage-sparing technique. It allows for the formation of the antihelical fold with the use of permanent sutures.[14] Furnas[15] described the use of sutures to reposition the concha against the mastoid periosteum. A combination of these techniques, with certain variations, has been used by surgeons in North America and across the world because of its simplicity and overall good results. Percutaneous or incisionless techniques have evolved from these cartilage-sparing techniques and are gaining in popularity.[12,16,17]

It is my opinion based on personal experience and observations that results obtained from cartilage-sparing techniques are more natural looking, require no or less skin undermining, and have a shorter operative time. The postoperative recovery is quicker and less complicated. The main disadvantage of these techniques is that it is harder to deal with very stiff cartilage as found in some adults, and the recurrence of the deformity may be higher.

There are various cartilage-cutting techniques that have been described and are used by surgeons. These techniques differ in approach (anterior, posterior, or both) and whether the cartilage is cut full thickness or partial thickness.[18–22]

The main advantages of some of these procedures are the ability to deal with stiff cartilage, the lack of permanent sutures in some cases, and a reduced rate of recurrence of the deformity. One great criticism of these techniques is that the results may look "operated" with sharp edges and a somewhat unnatural aesthetic result. The postoperative management of these patients is more protracted and requires more long-term splinting and bandaging. Revision surgery in these patients is more difficult due to the scarring encountered in the cut cartilage.

NEVES

I believe that the less a structure is traumatized, the lower the rate of complications. I avoid creating possible sharp areas where they are meant to be smooth. When I recreate the antihelical fold, I mainly use cartilage-sparing techniques, because the problem is lack of definition and not excess of cartilage. I do not see any advantage in excising or cutting the cartilage. The use of sutures allows sculpting the cartilaginous framework as desired. I start by recreating and defining the antihelical fold and then I set back the entire auricular complex. In cases of milder deformities, the use of 2 or 3 setback sutures in the right place allows the pinna to assume the ideal definition.

In patients with stronger and thicker cartilage, such as adult men, the suture technique on its own may lead to higher rates of relapse and revision surgery. In these cases, I like to weaken the

anterior surface of the cartilage at the level of the soon to be created antihelical fold. This, I believe, facilitates the creation of the fold and its long-term stability. I think that cutting the cartilage is disadvantageous so I create small subperichondrial tunnels along the anterior surface of the scapha and use a fine diamond rasp to reduce the cartilage strength in this area. This allows me to help the sutures define the fold, increase stability, and avoid the possibility of creating visible irregularities.

I do cut the cartilage in cases where the concha is very hypertrophic. This is performed in the area of transition between the antihelix and the concha. This is a hidden area of the ear, where the cuts are not visible and are not being used to recreate a fold but to excise extra cartilage and allow for better positioning of the pinna.

TASMAN

The goal of any otoplasty is a normal-appearing, inconspicuous auricle that does not attract the attention of the casual observer. Protruding ears do catch attention[23], but little is known about the effect of a nonprotruding but unnatural-appearing ear. Techniques that bring about a higher risk of trading one deformity, such as severe protrusion, for another, such as loss of natural appearance through surgery, should be viewed critically. I believe this is the case for cartilage-cutting techniques. Looking back on years of routinely using cartilage-cutting techniques, the Converse technique in particular, I have learned from my own mistakes and unfavorable outcomes from others. Not only do I attribute this to inexperience and technical errors, but also the technique per se (**Fig. 1**). As a rule, I try to avoid incisions at or around esthetically critical structures, such as the antihelical fold. I will, however, excise cartilage from a markedly hyperplastic bowl-shaped cavum concha, sparing the cavum conchae skin most of the time. To me, the decisive advantage of sparing the cartilage when recreating the antihelical fold is the reduced risk of creating a fold that appears unnatural or sharp. The main disadvantage, in rigid cartilage in particular, is the persistent recoil of the cartilage that may reduce the reliability of sutures, if not addressed by weakening the cartilage. Another advantage of cartilage-sparing techniques is that they are reversible, at least theoretically. Then, revising an undercorrection or overcorrection with the continuity of the antihelical cartilage intact is much easier that the same procedure with discontinuous cartilage. Sharp edges after folding incised cartilage may be impossible to correct entirely. Finally, in teaching settings, I find cartilage-sparing techniques easier to teach

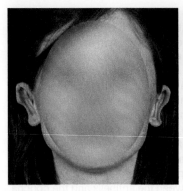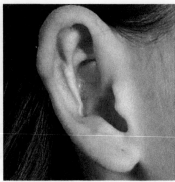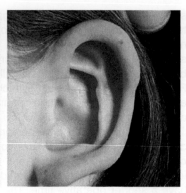

Fig. 1. Unfavorable outcome after a cartilage-splitting otoplasty. Both auricles show a persistent ear protrusion, a telephone ear deformity, and visible sharp edge irregularities with blanching of the skin overlying the sharp edges.

and safer in the hands of the less experienced surgeon.

Question 3: What is your preferred surgical technique when performing otoplasty? What are the indications and contraindications for this technique in your hands? If you do not perform your usual technique, what other techniques do you perform?

TASMAN

My preferred otoplasty technique is a combination of the Mustardé suture technique, with or without weakening of the anterior cartilaginous surface of the antihelical fold, in combination with a Furnas concha-mastoid suture (**Fig. 2**). Directing the concho-mastoid suture in a posteromedial direction reduces the risk of narrowing the external meatus and obviates resection of a cartilage crescent at the posterior circumference of the meatal entrance. If prominent, I also correct the ear lobe, with or without partial resection of the antitragus. In adults and in some children from the age of 12 onward, I prefer local anesthesia with xylocaine 1%, with adrenaline 1:200,000 without sedation. In 4 of 5 patients who do not present with very weak cartilage, I weaken the cartilage after infiltration of the anterior surface (**Fig. 3**). This has helped reduce the incidence of recurrences seen in patients with stiff cartilage in whom an isolated Mustardé technique had been used. This is the technique I use in the vast majority of my primary otoplasty patients. Gross anatomic variations or distortions due to previous surgery (see **Fig. 1**) contraindicate this approach. I have found this technique sufficiently versatile, quick, and safe to use in almost all patients with a hypoplastic antihelical fold with or without conchal hyperplasia and apostasis.

GANTOUS

My preferred surgical technique for the correction of prominauris is the incisionless otoplasty. I have been performing this procedure almost exclusively since 2006 and have become more comfortable with its versatility and lessened its limitations. The

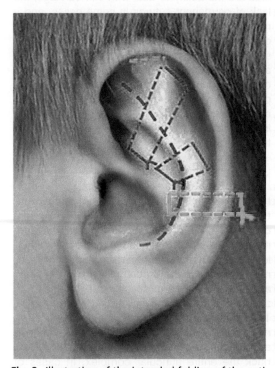

Fig. 2. Illustration of the intended folding of the antihelix (*red dashed line*), incision of the cartilage at the level of the free margin of the helix from the posterior surface of the auricle (*light blue dashed line*), area of skin elevation on the anterior auricular surface (*light blue shaded area*), 2 Mustardé sutures (*superior 2 blue dashed rectangles*), and a Furnas concha-mastoid suture (*lower dashed green rectangle and arrow*).

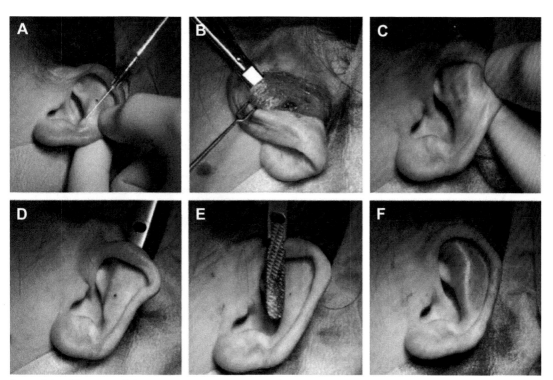

Fig. 3. (*A*) Infiltration of the posterior and anterior surfaces of the auricle with xylocaine 1% and adrenaline 1:200,000. (*B*) After the posterior surface of the auricular cartilage has been dissected, a 6-mm incision is made at the level of the free margin of the helix and parallel to the helix, from posterior to anterior. (*C, D*) The skin and the perichondrium are elevated from the anterior surface of the conchal cartilage at the desired location of the new antihelical fold. The dissection is carried down to the level of the external meatus. (*E*) A take-apart rasp (Medicon, Germany; blade number 4) is used to contour the anterior surface of the cartilage by pressing the rasp and cartilage between index finger and thumb. The surface of the cartilage is shaved off until the cartilage has the desired softness. Care is taken to take down as little cartilage as needed, using the full width of the rasp to avoid a sharp antihelical fold. (*F*) Intraoperative result after placing 1 of 2 Mustardé sutures.

anterior and posterior surfaces of the auricles are infiltrated with lidocaine with epinephrine 1:200,000 in all patients. A general anesthetic is used in children and straight local anesthesia in teenagers and adults. I use a 4-0 Ti-Cron or Mersilene suture with a $\frac{1}{2}$ Circle 1834-7D cutting edge needle (Anchor Products) and place percutaneous horizontal mattress sutures to recreate the antihelical fold, set back the concha, and reposition the ear lobe when needed. A 22-gauge hypodermic needle is used to score the scaphal cartilage percutaneously on its anterior surface along the soon to be recreated antihelical fold (**Fig. 4**, Video 1).

We looked at our results using this technique over a period of 8 years in both adults and children and found it a reliable and replicable operation with which consistently good outcomes could be obtained.[19] This technique can be used in almost all patients with prominent ears who wish to undergo an otoplasty (**Figs. 5** and **6**).

I find that patients with severe cup ear deformities where the pinna is reduced in size are harder to treat with this technique.

I have not had reliable results trying to correct Stahl ears with an incisionless approach. Adult patients who have very thick cartilage are warned that they need a thicker suture (3–0 Mersilene) and have a slightly higher rate of recurrence. In patients with excessively large conchal bowls, I resect some cartilage and use 2 or 3 conchomastoid sutures via an open approach (I do not resect skin and only elevate a limited skin flap still placing my antihelical sutures percutaneously). I find that I seldom have to do this, however.

NEVES

I divide my surgical approach into 2 different approaches depending on 2 distinct diagnoses: the absence of antihelical definition and the

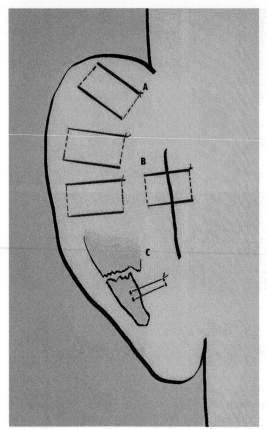

Fig. 4. The different sutures that can be used in an incisionless otoplasty. A, scaphal sutures for creation of the antihelix; B, concho-mastoid suture, and C, cauda helicis suture. (*Courtesy of* Andres Gantous, MD, Toronto, Ontario.)

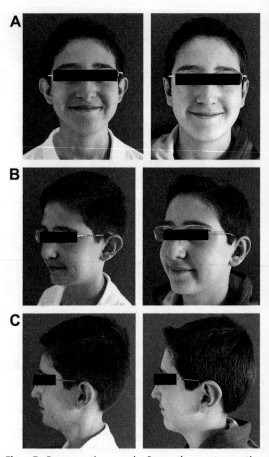

Fig. 5. Preoperative and 6-month postoperative photos of a young patient who underwent incisionless otoplasty.

overprojection of the concha. Both deformities can be in the same ear, in which case these 2 approaches can be easily combined.

In cases of absence of the antihelical fold, I use a suture technique. I start to draw the antihelix and decide where to put my sutures to achieve a natural slightly curved antihelix based on the principle described by Mustardé. I use 2 to 3 4-0 clear nylon horizontal mattress sutures, avoiding overcorrection of this compartment. My goal is just to create definition of the antihelix without hiding the helical rim. Care must be taken to include all the cartilage and perichondrium without having suture exposure under the skin. If the cartilage is thick and strong, especially in adults, I create a subperichondrial tunnel on the anterior surface of the ear over the antihelix to introduce a delicate diamond rasp to release tension and make the cartilage more pliable.

I then reposition the auricular framework with 2 or 3 setback sutures. The mastoid periosteum and the temporal fascia are exposed by removing

the soft tissues overlying them. A first stitch, clear 3-0 nylon, is placed through the conchal cartilage and the mastoid periosteum to bring the framework medially and posteriorly (avoiding distortion of the external acoustic meatus). Again care must be taken not to overcorrect by creating a C-shaped deformity on the frontal view. The more the medial third of the concha is brought medially, the more the upper helix, as well as the lobule, may lateralize. A second suture is placed from the posterior surface of the fossa triangularis to the temporal fascia. This suture helps harmonize the natural curvature of the helix and helps stabilize the ear further. Less frequently, I place a third suture in the lower part of the concha (form concha to mastoid) to help control the overprotected lobule.

When I have an overprojected concha with a well-formed antihelix, I use the technique that I call the "pillars concept" (**Fig. 7**). Think of the support framework of the pinna as a bridge with a wall under it. This oval bridge based on the antihelix

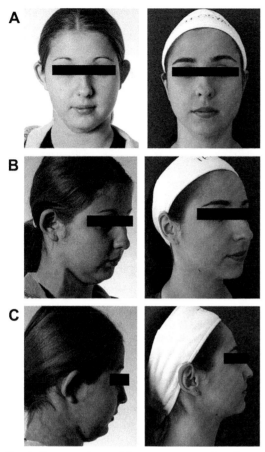

Fig. 6. Preoperative and 8-year postoperative photos of a teenage patient who underwent incisionless otoplasty.

starts as a superior pillar, with its base settled between the spine of the helix and the end of the inferior crus of the antihelix, and an inferior pillar, which is stabilized on the incisura intertragica. It is because of this concept that the concha (the wall under the bridge) can be harvested and the rest of the framework (the bridge) stays in the same position. But if these pillars are cut, interrupting the forces that keep the bridge in suspension, the whole structure falls posteriorly (**Fig. 8**). This allows for a complete repositioning of the ear where it is wanted while maintaining the natural and well-defined antihelix (**Fig. 9**).

I first started using this technique with complete conchal cartilage excision, but this only makes sense if the cartilage is needed for grafting, for example, in a concomitant rhinoplasty. If I do not need to harvest the conchal cartilage, I spare it and use 2 other techniques to bring the conchal height to its desired position. I divide the antihelix from the concha and I mark the excess concha to be removed. The anterior skin flap must be elevated up to the external auditory canal to redistribute the skin over a smaller concha. The 2 cartilaginous borders are brought together and sutured along the cut edge to avoid a posterior displacement of the antihelix and a visible step deformity (**Fig. 10**). In patients with bigger conchae, when the excess concha is cut, the 2 cut edges are asymmetric, the conchal edge smaller than the antihelical edge. This can make the suturing of the 2 cartilaginous edges tricky. So an alternative is to bring the all concha posteriorly and suture it

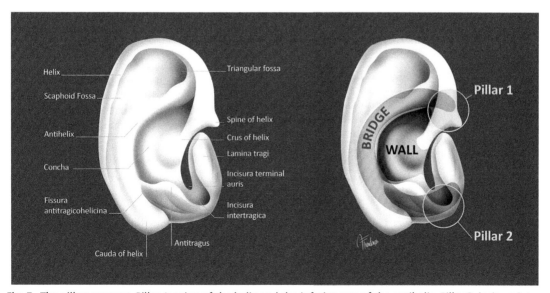

Fig. 7. The pillars concept. Pillar 1: spine of the helix and the inferior crus of the antihelix. Pillar 2: incisura intertragica. (*Courtesy of* Jose Carlos Neves, MD, Lisboa, Portugal.)

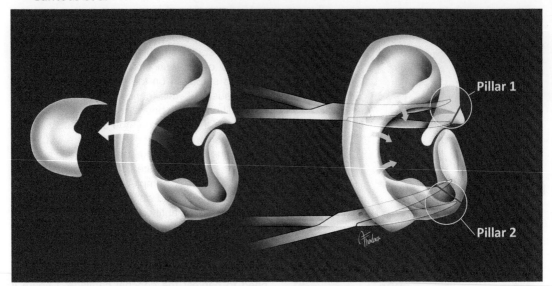

Fig. 8. Hypertrophic concha: concha excised and the pillars cut. (*Courtesy of* Jose Carlos Neves, MD, Lisboa, Portugal.)

A

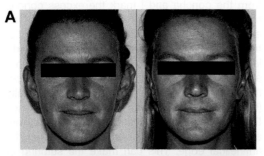

B

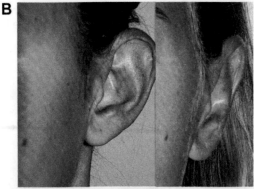

C

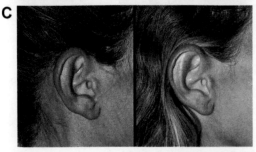

Fig. 9. Preoperative and postoperative photos of a patient treated with the pillars concept technique. No antihelical sutures used.

to the mastoid periosteum allowing the rest of the framework to fall posteriorly to the desired position (**Fig. 11**). Care must be taken to assess the size of the concha when it is being set back. I frequently cut a slice of concha before suturing it to the mastoid to avoid a visible deformity postoperatively. In all these conchal hypertrophy approaches, a bolster suture is placed to prevent a hematoma under the anterior skin flap. I use a 2-0 silk suture for 48 hours.

Question 4: How do you deal with the prominent ear lobe?

GANTOUS

Ear lobe repositioning has always been a challenge for surgeons. I do not find that the traditional skin excision is a reliable technique for correcting this anomaly. I have been using the technique described by Fritsch where the cauda helicis is percutaneously detached inferiorly and then repositioned with a percutaneous suture, bringing the ear lobe to the plane of the scapha.

TASMAN

Most of the time, a protrusion of the lobule that persists after folding the antihelix and rotating the cavum can be dealt with by a posterior excision of skin and subcutaneous tissue. It may be necessary to dissect and reduce the cartilaginous antitragus. Variations include dissecting the lobule between and parallel to the anterior and posterior skin surfaces and placing a traction suture between the posterior half of the dissected tragus caudally and the conchal cartilage more cranially,

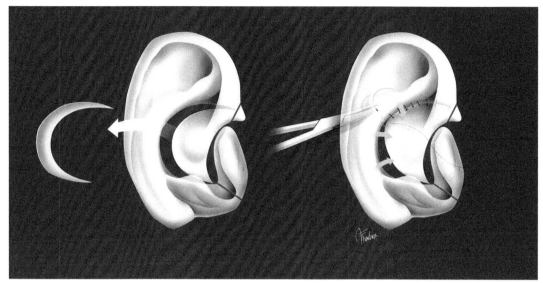

Fig. 10. Hypertrophic concha: only excess cartilage excised. (*Courtesy of* Jose Carlos Neves, MD, Lisboa, Portugal.)

pulling the tragus inward.[24] A Y-to-V plasty, as described by Weerda,[25] is another time-tested technique.

NEVES

Sometimes I create an apparent prominent ear lobe when the middle setback sutures are too tight, creating a C-shaped deformity. So, first, care must be directed to avoid this undesired effect. It is important to keep in mind that overtightening of the middle third of the ear is not the ideal.

The aim is to spread the forces throughout the 3 thirds of the ear framework. Using a concho-mastoid suture in the lower third of the concha not only helps harmonize the natural curvature of the helix-antihelix relation but also avoids the prominent lobule.

In mild cases of ear lobe prominence, I perform an elliptical skin excision with direct closure.

Most often, I use an elliptical-shaped 4-0 clear nylon suture, passing it through the soft tissues of the lobule, halfway between the antitragus and the caudal border of the lobule and the concha.

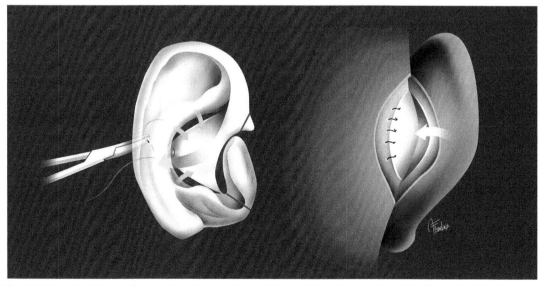

Fig. 11. Hypertrophic concha: sparing the concha and the cartilage being sutured to the mastoid periosteum. (*Courtesy of* Jose Carlos Neves, MD, Lisboa, Portugal.)

If this suture is too tight, a cartilaginous deformity may be visible along the antitragus.

In more rare cases, if the cauda helicis is too overprojected, it can be partially removed and one of other techniques, described previously, applies.

Question 5: How do you manage your otoplasty patients postoperatively?

TASMAN

After closure of the posterior skin incision, typically with a fast-absorbing 5-0 monofilament suture, a loose circular head dressing is applied and left in place for 18 hours to 24 hours. Most patients prefer to remove the dressing themselves or have it removed by parents or partners on the day after surgery. No dressing is worn during daytime thereafter. Wearing a headband at night for 2 weeks is advised. Antibiotics or topical treatments are not prescribed. The patients are handed out a supply of nonsteroidal anti-inflammatory drugs for the first 24 hours and instructed to contact the surgeon's staff should pain persist or reappear after 24 hours. Patients are seen 4 weeks to 8 weeks after surgery. The prospect of receiving the preoperative photos, the computer simulation, and pictures of the actual outcome helps motivate the patients for a follow-up appointment.

NEVES

I perform otoplasty as an outpatient procedure. A dressing is placed for 48 hours. It consists of Vaseline-impregnated wool strings conformed over the newly shaped and positioned cartilage and a cotton wool bolster over the ears secured in position by a gauze or flannel roll.

If an antihemorrhagic bolster mattress suture is used and if there is no sign of hematoma or bleeding, it is also removed at the same time. I close the skin with 5-0 Vicryl rapid, so it does not need to be removed; this is significantly important in children.

After 2 days, patients return to their normal activities without any dressing during the day.

I ask patients to apply Vaseline ointment on the posterior skin for the first week to keep the wound moist.

For a period of no less than 2 months, I ask patients to sleep with a headband to avoid unexpected trauma. It is especially important when the position and the shape of the cartilage depend on sutures. When the pillars concept approach is used, theoretically, there is no chance for a relapse once the mechanisms of support that keep the concha overprotected are cut. Patients follow-up

in the office at 1 week postoperatively and then at 1 month, 3 months, 6 months, and 12 months.

GANTOUS

Children are managed with light otoplasty dressing consisting of cotton soaked in mineral oil in the preuricular and postauricular areas, fluffed gauze, and a gauze or flannel bandage wrapped around the head. This is kept in place for 24 hours, and the parents remove it at home. Teenagers and adults usually do not require any bandaging unless requested. Patients start washing the ears gently with soapy water the day after the procedure and use a bacteriostatic ointment twice a day over the needle holes for a week. Analgesia is managed with acetaminophen, ibuprofen, or oral narcotics if needed. No antibiotics are used. Patients wear an athletic headband at night for at least 2 weeks. They are told that they can wear it during the day if they desire. They are seen in follow-up at 1 week and 1 month postoperatively and then at 6 months.

Question 6: What are the sociocultural and technical considerations in performing otoplasty in nonwhite patients?

GANTOUS

I do not believe that there are any technical considerations that should differ in treating nonwhite patients when performing otoplasty. The goals of the operation and the technique used are going to be the same in most cases. The possibility of keloid formation and/or hypertrophic scarring has to be taken into account, however.

The one thing that I have encountered in my practice is the negative reaction of parents of Asian descent when I have touched on the possibility of performing an otoplasty in their child. Many Asian cultures believe that large ears are a sign of good luck and/or wisdom. Whether this comes from the large ears of the Buddha or from ancient face reading is unknown.[26]

Question 7: How have your techniques in this area changed over the past 5 years?

GANTOUS

I have become more comfortable with the incisionless technique and begun to address a wider range of prominent ear deformities. I have modified some of the suturing techniques to get more consistent results. In particular, I have changed how I place the concho-mastoid percutaneous suture (when I need to use it) to get a bigger bite of the mastoid periosteum and a larger area suture contact with the conchal cartilage (**Fig. 12**).

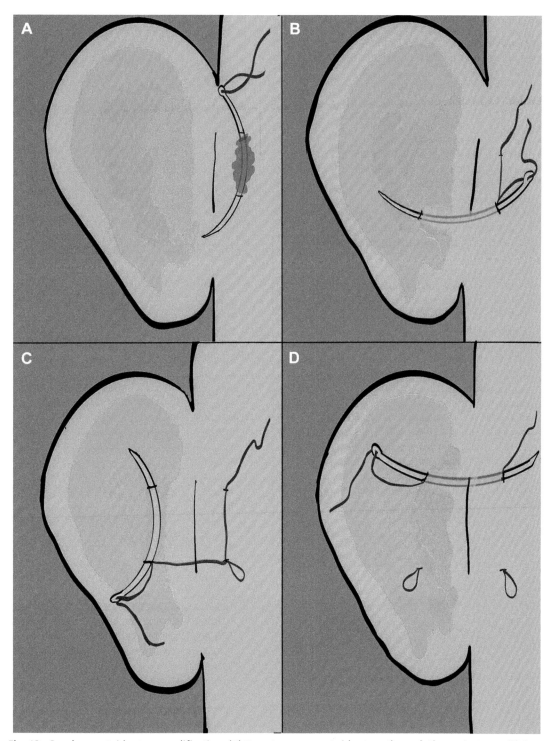

Fig. 12. Concho-mastoid suture modification. (*A*) Percutaneous mastoid suture through the periosteum. (*B*) Post-auricular subcutaneous pass. (*C*) Pass through auricular cartilage. (*D*) Postauricular subcutaneous pass. (*Courtesy of* Andres Gantous, MD, Toronto, Ontario.)

SUPPLEMENTARY DATA

Supplementary data related to this article can be found online at https://doi.org/10.1016/j.fsc.2017.12.010.

REFERENCES

1. Adamson PA, Strecker HD. Otoplasty techniques. Facial Plast Surg 1995;11:284–300.
2. Matsuo K, Hayashi R, Kiyono M, et al. Nonsurgical correction of congenital auricular deformities. Clin Plast Surg 1990;17(2):383–95.
3. Byrd HS, Langevin CJ, Ghidone LA. Ear molding in newborn infants with auricular deformities. Plast Reconstr Surg 2010;126(4):1191–200.
4. Macgregor FC. Ear deformities: social and psychological implications. Clin Plast Surg 1978;5(3):347–50.
5. Kurozumi N, Ono S, Ishida H. Nonsurgical correction of a congenital lop ear deformity by splinting with Reston foam. Br J Plast Surg 1982;35:181–2.
6. Muraoka M, Nakai Y, Ohashi Y, et al. Tape attachment therapy for correction of congenital malformations of the auricle: clinical and experimental studies. Laryngoscope 1985;95:167–76.
7. Tan ST, Abramson DL, MacDonald DM, et al. Molding therapy for infants with deformational auricular anomalies. Ann Plast Surg 1997;38:263–8.
8. Pawar SS, Koch CA, Murakami C. Treatment of prominent ears and otoplasty: a contemporary review. JAMA Facial Plast Surg 2015;17(6):449–54.
9. Doft MA, Goodkind AB, Diamond S, et al. The newborn butterfly project: a shortened treatment protocol for ear molding. Plast Reconstr Surg 2015;135(3):577e–83e.
10. Leclère FM, Vogt PM, Casoli V, et al. Laser-assisted cartilage reshaping for protruding ears: a review of the clinical applications. Laryngoscope 2015;125(9):2067–71.
11. Leclère FM, Mordon S, Alcolea J, et al. 1064-nm Nd:YAG laser- assisted cartilage reshaping for treating ear protrusions. Laryngoscope 2015;125(11):2461–7.
12. Fritsch MH. Incisionless otoplasty. Laryngoscope 1995;105(5 pt 3 suppl 70):1–11.
13. Mehta S, Gantous A. Incisionless otoplasty: a reliable and replicable technique for the correction of prominauris. JAMA Facial Plast Surg 2014;16(6):414–8.
14. Mustarde JC. The correction of prominent ears using simple mattress sutures. Br J Plast Surg 1963;16:170–8.
15. Furnas D. Correction of prominent ears by conchamastoid sutures. Plast Reconstr Surg 1968;42(3):189–93.
16. Fritsch MH. Incisionless otoplasty. Otolaryngol Clin North Am 2009;42:1199–208.
17. Haytoglu S, Haytoglu TG, Bayar Muluk N, et al. Comparison of two incisionless techniques for prominent ears in children. Int J Pediatr Otorhinolaryngol 2015;79(4):504–10.
18. Converse JM, Nigro A, Wilson FA, et al. A technique for surgical correction of lop ears. Plast Reconstr Surg 1955;15(5):411–8.
19. Pitanguy Y, Rebello C. Ansiform ears correction by "island" technique. Acta Chir Plast 1962;4:267–77.
20. Jost J. Atlas of aesthetic plastic surgery. Paris: Masson; 1975.
21. Obadia D, Quilichini J, Huisinger V, et al. Cartilage splitting without stitches: technique and outcomes. JAMA Facial Plast Surg 2013;15(6):428–33.
22. Stenström SJ, Heftner J. The Stenström otoplasty. Clin Plast Surg 1978;5(3):465–70.
23. Litschel R, Majoor J, Tasman AJ. Effect of protruding ears on visual fixation time and perception of personality. JAMA Facial Plast Surg 2015;17(3):183–9.
24. Sadick H, Artinger VM, Haubner F, et al. Correcting the lobule in otoplasty using the fillet technique. JAMA Facial Plast Surg 2014;16(1):49–54.
25. Weerda H, editor. Surgery of the auricle: tumorstrauma-defects-abnormalities. Thieme Publishers; 2004. p. 137.
26. Wong FTC, Soo G, Ng WP, et al. Implications of Chinese face reading on the aesthetic sense. Arch Facial Plast Surg 2010;12(4):218–21.

Lip Augmentation

Louis M. DeJoseph, MD[a],*, Anurag Agarwal, MD[b], Timothy M. Greco, MD[c]

KEYWORDS

• Lip augmentation • Lip injection • Lip surgery • Aging lips • Lip implants • Lip enhancement

KEY POINTS

• Cosmetic assessment and patient selection for lip augmentation is important for success.
• Different techniques include injection, surgery, implants, and laser resurfacing.
• Recognizing and managing complications is paramount to anyone performing lip augmentation.

Panel discussion

1. What is your nonsurgical method or technique for volumizing?
2. What complications have you observed with lip rejuvenation and what is your management strategy?
3. What surgical methods do you like for lip enhancement?
4. What technique do you use to resurface lines around the lips or perioral area?
5. What is your personal view on the aesthetic enhancement of the lips and recent trends you have observed?
6. How have your techniques in this area changed over the last 5 years?

Question 1: What is your nonsurgical method or technique for volumizing?

DeJoseph

The aging process of the face involves many structures including the bony skeleton, fat, soft tissue, and skin.[1] The lip in particular is a focal point of beauty on the face; pouty, full lips are synonymous with youth. Loss of these features attributes to the overall aging appearance of the face.[2] My personal technique with nonsurgical volumization to the lips starts with an evaluation of the aging issues at hand. I examine for symmetry, movement, overall shape, and volume. This examination is done during the idle conversation of how the patient's vacation was or how their children doing. Examination of the lips in this dynamic habitat tells you a lot about what needs to be done.

I approach lip volumization in a simple 3-pronged approach: (1) structure, (2) volume, or (3) both. A lip that needs purely structure is one where some highlight and "pop" at the vermillion border is all that is needed. Volume is adequate and highlight is needed. In this instance, I inject a hyaluronic acid product with a 30x ½ inch needle along the lip border about 2 mm inside the vermillion border. I do this along the entire length of the upper and lower lips. I find there is a space there where the filler flows and allows a smooth even contour. I also routinely put a small amount in the philtral columns to add highlight to the cupid's bow area. Less is more in here. In the second instance, the lip has a nice shape and structure, but is missing a healthy, youthful volume. For this, I use the same product and syringe as above, but place the product at the wet–dry border of the lip or where they touch in closed repose. For the upper lip, I only inject the outer thirds and not

---

Disclosure Statement: The authors have nothing to disclose.
[a] Department Otolaryngology Head and Neck Surgery, Emory University, Atlanta, GA, USA; [b] Private Practice, 1175, Creekside, Pkwy#100, Naples, FL 34108, USA; [c] Perelman School of Medicine, University of Pennsylvania School of Medicine, Philadelphia, PA, USA
* Corresponding author. Premier Image Cosmetic & Laser Surgery, 6085 Barfield Road, Suite 100, Atlanta, GA 30328.
E-mail address: LDejoseph@premierimage.com

the middle. I feel this keeps a more natural architecture and avoids the upper lip worm look secondary to the loss of the midline architecture at the philtrum. The lower lip is injected along its entire length, with an emphasis on the middle third to add a slight pout. I preferentially fill the lower lip to keep the balance and prevent the popularized large upper lip. The last scenario is one where structure at the vermillion and volume in the lip body is needed. Here, I combine these techniques to achieve what I want. I always err on conservative filling because you can always add more. Caution is warranted in the aged, thin-lipped patient who wants a larger lip. In this instance, where the upper lip almost disappears, it is hard to get more red to show. These patients often end up with an anteriorly displaced lip instead of a beautiful one. It is important to discuss this in the assessment and to communicate clearly with the patient the limitation of injection.

AGARWAL

Full lips have long been considered aesthetically attractive, sensual, and youthful. Patients often seek volumization of their lips, which may be thin as a baseline genetic trait or may progressively thin as part of the well-described aging process. The initial physician assessment of any new patient must include a thorough understanding of the patient's aesthetic ideals and goals, as well as examination and analysis of his or her lips and facial proportions. In the vast majority of cases, these patients seek initial and often ongoing treatment with nonsurgical methods. It is incumbent on the treating provider to recognize the limitations in volumization that can be achieved when the patient presents with extremely thin lips at baseline with limited vermilion show and/or a long cutaneous upper lip. All too often, patients have an unrealistic expectation of their outcome based on photographs of models, pop icons, or friends whose baseline lip fullness and shape vary greatly from their own. It is important to explain how much augmentation can be achieved before treatment to avoid having a disappointed patient.

Injectable hyaluronic acid filler allows for immediate results with low down time, generally a 4- to 8-month longevity, and reversibility. Because of the thin nature of the vermilion mucosa overlying the orbicularis oris muscle, injections are generally placed at the deepest aspect of the mucosa, just above and sometimes within the orbicularis muscle. This is done to avoid visible bumps and nodules. I prefer using the smooth consistency gel, JUVEDERM Ultra XC (Allergan, Inc., Dublin, Ireland), which extrudes easily and in a consistent manner. The retrograde injection technique is used, with fanning in certain cases. Although my injection pattern varies based on the patient's anatomy and goals, the following is my most common pattern of injection for volumizing the lips: After the application of topical anesthetic cream for 15 minutes, the filler is injected in primarily 2 zones, described by Jacono[3] as the subvermilion and peristomal zones. I avoid injecting the vermilion border at the white roll because, in my opinion, this can create an unnaturally prominent ridge that looks artificial (the exception to this is when I am treating the senile lip with vertical lip rhytids using a very small amount of JUVEDERM Volbella XC along the vermilion border/white roll and isolated vertical lip rhytids[4]). Injection of the subvermilion zone is performed first along the length of the upper and lower lip, following the contours of the cupid's bow to preserve its native shape. Because most patients desire lateral lip fullness, I often inject the lateral subvermilion and peristomal zones through 1 or 2 needle puncture sites, using the fanning technique to evenly distribute the product. It is imperative to develop a consistent pattern of extrusion and monitor amounts delivered during injection to avoid asymmetrical deposition of product from side to side. For those individuals seeking more pout and/or dramatic augmentation, I subsequently inject the natural prominences lateral to the midline of the upper and lower lip, known as the "upper and lower lip tubercles."[5] Finally, after visual inspection, I manually check for symmetry using my thumb and index finger on each side of the patient's lips with gentle pressure. If I can feel a deficiency in one area but cannot see a deficiency, I add a small aliquot of filler to the deficient area to achieve palpable symmetry.

Because edema sets in relatively quickly, it is critical to inject similar volumes from side to side, in a stepwise fashion as each area is treated (barring any baseline lip asymmetries that are being corrected). I rarely inject more than 1 mL of filler in a treatment session because I find that the incidence of asymmetry and/or bumps increases with higher volumes of injection in a given treatment session. For those patients seeking more dramatic augmentation, I encourage a second syringe to be administered in a delayed fashion 2 weeks later.

GRECO

To appropriately volumize the lips, it is important to understand the embryology of these structures. The upper lip is formed by 3 embryologic units and the lower lip is formed from 2.[6] Also, understanding certain aesthetic norms of the lips is important. The upper lip should embody 40% of the vermilion show on front view and the lower lip 60%. Also, the lip show anteriorly can be expressed in using the phi ratio as 1:1.618 with 1 being the upper lip and 1.618 being the lower lip. The upper lip should project 2 mm in front of the lower lip on profile. The tubercles of the upper and lower lip should fit together aesthetically and gently, like pieces of a delicate puzzle with the central tubercle of the upper lip nestled between a subtle cleft found centrally in the lower lip. Also, evaluate the patient's occlusion before injecting the lips. Retrognathia gives the upper lip pseudoaugmentation and this feature needs to be taken into account before injecting. When volumizing the lips, I prefer to use a cannula and provide a regional block to the lips so as not to distort the natural anatomy of the lips from direct injection of local anesthetic. The cannula is placed at the oral commissure after an entrance has been made with a slightly larger needle. The cannula that I most frequently use for my lip augmentation is a 27-gauge 1.5-inch cannula and a 25-gauge 0.5-inch entrance needle. This is made just outside the pink portion of the oral commissure. Once there is sufficient portal of entry for the cannula, the cannula is advanced just inside the pink portion of the upper lip and advanced along the vermilion border to create a crisp border for the purposes of placing lip liner and also to prevent lipstick bleed. This technique is a great way of taking care of those deep lip rhytids that extend into the vermilion.

Next, the cannula is advanced to the Cupid's bow and the unilateral side of the Cupid's bow is augmented to the midline. The philtral column can also be augmented by realigning the philtral column by using the noninjecting hand to align the column with the vermillion border. The cannula is then withdrawn, but remains inside the lip. The tubercles are then augmented with product in such a manner that a gentle enhancement is performed by creating a delicate mound, as opposed to a lump. Three tubercles are augmented on the upper lip, secondary to the embryology of the lip. Next, if lip eversion is necessary, the cannula is directed posterior to the orbicularis oris submucosally in the region of the frenulum and a small bolus of product deposited. The lower lip is enhanced using a similar technique. The vermillion border is enhanced first across its entire length. Next, the 2 tubercles of the lower lip are enhanced being careful to maintain a subtle central cleft. Eversion is accomplished using the same technique used on the upper lip and placing product submucosally and just anterior to the frenulum. A small depo is placed by a linear threading technique this helps to create lip eversion. The products used for lip augmentation with minimally invasive techniques are usually a low viscosity hyaluronic acid (Juvederm Ultra) or a small particle hyaluronic acid (Restylane). Gentle massage is accomplished with Aquaphor to avoid lumps. The amount of product injected is monitored carefully throughout the procedure to make sure that equal amounts are placed when the lips are symmetric before injection and appropriate asymmetric amounts are injected when there is asymmetry of the lips before injection.

Question 2: What complications have you observed with lip rejuvenation and what is your management strategy?

DeJoseph

The most common adverse events I have witnessed from lip rejuvenation are bruising and swelling. These effects can be expected on almost all patients to some extent with these maneuvers, but education of the front end is paramount to patient satisfaction. I will have patents stop all nonsteroidal antiinflammatory drugs, vitamins, omega 3, or blood thinning agents 2 weeks if possible before lip procedures. Swelling can be a wildcard to lip rejuvenation and must be discussed before the procedure. I ask patients what they have going on socially and at work for the next several days because the swelling can be prohibitive. Management of swelling begins at the time of injection with slow, low-pressure injection. Then minimal and gentle manipulation of the lip to smooth the filler. I have found that vigorous massage of the lips afterward can lead to more intense swelling. Choice of filler can also play a role; some products intrinsically swell more than others. Finally, ice packs are offered immediately after treatment. Rarely, the swelling is extreme, or longer lasting. In these cases, patients are seen in the office and if deemed necessary a tapering steroid dose is given to abate the swelling.

Herpes simplex virus infection has come up and can surface in a patient with no prior history. I treat these infections with a 10-day course of acyclovir. I do not routinely pretreat with antivirals for lip injections, but I do prescribe prophylactic antiviral medication for surgical lip procedures.

Asymmetry is a common complaint with lip fillers and easily handled with additional filler to correct or hyaluronidase to adjust the filler present.[7]

Last, I have witness and treated vascular compromise from injection to the lips. This is seen in **Fig. 1**, which shows a patient sent to me after 3 days after lip injection with hyaluronic

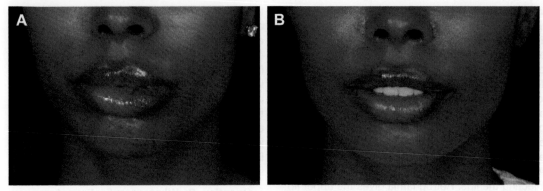

Fig. 1. (A) Patient 3 days after hyaluronic acid injection elsewhere. (B) Three weeks after treatment with hyaluronidase to area.

acid. Anyone injecting this area or the face should know how to recognize this and treat it swiftly. Blanching of the lip and pain have been the most common signs in my experience. Treatment consists of high doses of hyaluronidase (ie, hundreds of units). Other adjuncts include aspirin administration, nitro paste, vigorous massage, and warm compresses. Of the cases I have treated, all have recovered with no sequelae. If the lip does not improve and impending tissue loss is noted, hyperbaric oxygen therapy is another useful step.[8]

AGARWAL

Complications from lip rejuvenation can be broken down into those arising from injectable nonsurgical treatment, versus those arising from surgical management. Complications from JUVEDERM Ultra XC injections are extremely rare. I have observed asymmetry once the edema resolves (treated with additional filler injection usually 2 weeks after initial injection), herpetic outbreak (treated with antivirals), and bumps from superficial injection. Bumps can be minimized by injecting in the deep mucosa or just within the superficial fibers of the orbicularis muscle. However, the greatest challenge lies in those patients who have had numerous prior injectable treatments of the lips. Fibrosis can cause filler to travel to unintended locations within the lips. This is instantly visible and exacerbated by excess extrusion force by the injector. When treating these types of patients, it is imperative to inject slowly, visualize the path of the filler, and to cease injecting immediately if the product travels beyond the intended location. I use digital massage more aggressively with these patients to try to disperse the product more evenly. If a bump is persistent within the lip and visible after 2 weeks, I inject the area with hyaluronidase conservatively.

My initial surgical lip augmentation of choice approximately 7 to 12 years ago was autologous sternocleidomastoid muscle and fascia graft insertion.[9] This technique offered a 20% to 25% increase in vermilion show and approximately a 1-mm increase in lip projection at 2 years and longer from baseline. This was most commonly performed at the same time as cervicofacial rhytidectomy but also as a standalone procedure. However, because it required intravenous anesthesia, many patients would avoid this option when seeking surgical lip rejuvenation as an isolated procedure. In addition, although the results demonstrated longevity, there were occasional asymmetries that required follow-up treatment, including further augmentation with injectable fillers. The greatest complication with this technique was the long-term substantial volume loss that occurred despite using sizable grafts at initial implantation. Patients were often happy 6 months postoperatively, but then disappointed with further reduction in volume over time as they expected a more "permanent" result.

In 2008, I began using the Perma Facial implant (Surgisil, L.L.P., Plano, TX) for permanent lip augmentation. Because these implants are symmetric in shape and can be inserted under local anesthesia in the office, they have become my surgical lip augmentation treatment of choice. The vast majority of patients on whom I have performed this technique have been very satisfied. However, I have observed 2 types of complications with these implants: One is superficial placement and visibility of the lateral tapered ends of the implant in the lower lip. This is due to the tendency to begin the submucosal tunnel too superficially near the oral commissure incisions. I have had to remove the implant, create a new deeper tunnel beginning at the oral commissure incision, and then replace the implant. The second complication I have observed is 1 case of capsular contracture, which was fortunately recognized early during the process as limited mouth opening and horizontal shortening/tightness of the lips. I manually stretched the patient's lips and encouraged the patient to vigorously massage the lips and perform lip stretching exercises. The contracture partially improved and the patient did not wish to have the implants removed. The inventors of this implant, Dr Peter Raphael and Dr Ryan Harris, use Accolate to treat capsular contracture,[10] but I have no experience with this approach. Since having the 1 case of capsular contracture in 2009, I have modified my postoperative instructions to have the patient begin mouth stretching exercises during the second week after the procedure. There have been no cases of dehiscence and no further cases of capsular contracture since this modification.

GRECO

I have found that, since converting to the cannula, the amount of complications and their severity has dramatically decreased when using hyaluronic acid fillers for lip augmentation. The most common complication that I encounter is swelling, which can be easily resolved with application of ice, having the patient maintain head of bed position while resting, and avoiding significant exercise for 24 hours after the injection. Since the transition to cannula, I have not encountered any ischemic episodes, nor have I encountered any hematomas. I have encountered an occasional lump that has occurred when seeing the patient back in 2 weeks. This is usually treated initially with massage. If for some reason resolution is not accomplished with massage, a small amount of Hylenex (hyaluronidase) can be injected into the raised area. Discretion has to be used when injecting Hylenex because you do not want to create a deformity in the lip because of overdissolving of the hyaluronic acid filler. No other complications have been encountered.

Question 3: What surgical methods do you like for lip enhancement?

DeJoseph

My 2 favorite surgical methods for lip enhancement are implantation and lifting. Lip implantation to add volume is ideal in the younger patient who desires a more permanent result. The method I use most commonly is with a Perma Lip silicone implant (Surgisil, L.L.P.) **Figs. 2** and **3** show before and after volumization with these implant techniques. This procedure is done under local anesthesia with upper and lower lip blocks if both lips are being augmented. Next, under obvious sterile technique, a small incision is placed in the commissures and a submucosal pocket is developed in the lip at the wet/dry border with a small iris scissors. A pearl here is to make sure the mucosal depth of the pocket is uniform across the lip or the implant may be visible when the patients smiles. Next, a curved tendon passer is placed through the pocket and brought out the other side. Care is taken to measure the lip beforehand along the wet/dry border to properly size the implant. My opinion is to err on more length to ensure the ends are not palpable and extend the full length to the commissures. The implant is then grasped at one end and pulled through the lip till until both ends are exposed. The implant is then centered and the ends are allowed to be released under the mucosa. The lower lip is implanted in the same manner via the same incisions if needed. The commissure incisions are then closed with chromic suture. If I am performing a rhytidectomy at the same sitting and a superficial muscular aponeurotic system (SMAS) is being removed, I have recycled this instead of the silicone implants into the lips for volume using this method for placement.

Last, when I encounter a patient with a thin upper lip who wants more red show, I like to perform a gull wing subnasal lip lift. I conceptualize

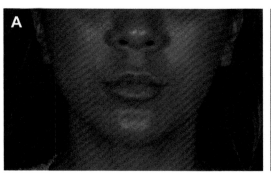
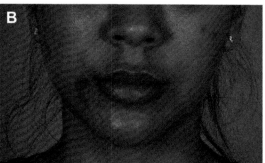

Fig. 2. (*A*) Before soft silicone implant in upper and lower lips. (*B*) Six months after soft silicone implant in upper and lower lips.

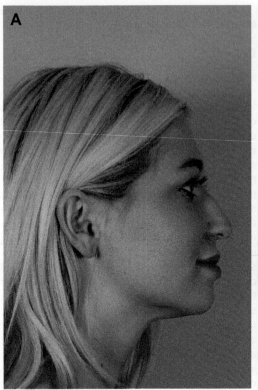 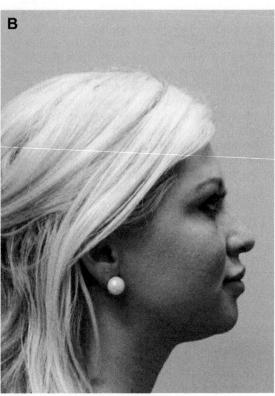

Fig. 3. (*A*) Silicone implants in lip before. (*B*) Silicone implants in lip after.

this as a blepharoplasty for the upper lip, because it should be performed with the same level of care and accuracy. A gull wing–like incision is designed in the subnasal area hugging the base of the collumela, entering the sill laterally, and then finally ending at the alar crease. A measuring caliper is then used to measure the amount of tissue to be removed and a mirror image is drawn below the initial site. This averages between 4 and 6 mm of skin. The incisions are made with a 15 blade scalpel and the skin is removed. I only undermine 1 to 2 mm of the lower incision to allow slight eversion with closure. The skin is then closed with 5-0 PDS suture in a buried deep dermal fashion and then a 5-0 nylon is used in a running subcuticular fashion and loped at the ends. This is removed in 5 days. These are my 2 main techniques for surgical enhancement of the lips.

AGARWAL

For those individuals with a normal length to their cutaneous upper lip, I perform lip augmentation using Perma Facial implants. These soft, malleable, silicone implants can be placed in the office with local anesthetic only or in conjunction with other surgical procedures performed with intravenous anesthesia. The implants are highly resistant to infection. They do not restrict the mobile lips because they are nonporous and do not allow tissue ingrowth. Patients do not experience any restriction in smiling, chewing, talking, or kissing and can only feel the implants when palpated with their fingers. They are counseled to expect some shifting of the implant from side to side.

Surgical pearls when placing Perma Facial implants (available in 3-, 4-, and 5-mm diameters) include the following:

- Avoid placing a 5-mm implant in an individual with thin lips. Otherwise, the outline of the implant may be visible because of aggressive distension of the mucosa.
- Begin the submucosal tunnel near the oral commissure incisions at the appropriate depth, rather than beginning too superficial. This step limits the visibility of the tapered ends of the implants.
- Measure the oral commissure to oral commissure distance carefully with the mouth slightly open, at the wet/dry junction of the lips. This step will allow appropriate horizontal sizing of the implants. Avoid using implants that are too short lest the end of the implant begins to be visible as it pushes against the mucosa well shy of the commissure.

- Keep the submucosal tunnel at a uniform depth while performing the dissection. Use visual and tactile assessments of tunnel depth when the curved passer is in place. If a portion of the tunnel is dissected too superficially, the implant will be visible at that location through the mucosa, especially when the patient smiles.
- Begin postoperative lip stretching exercises during the second week after surgery to minimize capsular contracture and lip restriction.

For those individuals with an excessively long cutaneous lip in conjunction with thin lips, I recommend a subnasal lip lift initially, followed by Perma Facial implants to the lips in a staged fashion. I stage this procedure because a subnasal lip lift causes external rotation of the upper lip, which increases upper lip vermilion show, thereby changing the ratio of upper to lower lip vermilion show. I prefer to allow 3 months for the lip to heal and swelling to resolve before taking measurements for Perma Facial implant sizing. The main complication that I have seen from a subnasal lip lift has been asymmetry of the apex of the cupid's bow from side to side. Meticulous measurements and markings before infiltration of a local anesthetic are the best way to avoid this complication. If it occurs, a revision lip lift is performed to elevate the side of the cupid's bow, which is lower. Only once symmetry has been satisfactorily achieved do I then proceed to place Perma Facial implants in these patients.

If a patient is not interested in having a foreign substance in their lips, or if they start off with a baseline asymmetry in lip size from side to side, then I recommend autologous sternocleidomastoid muscle and fascia grafts to the lips.[9] The patient must be counseled appropriately as to the degree of subtle long-term augmentation that can be achieved. Persistent fullness has been demonstrated at 2 years postoperatively. The grafts can be contoured to be fuller on one side to try to improve baseline asymmetries. This maneuver is not possible with the symmetrically shaped Perma Facial implants, the placement of which may preserve or even accentuate baseline lip asymmetries. The downside to the autologous grafts has been gradual resorption and/or potential for asymmetry owing to differential resorption from side to side.

GRECO

There are 2 methods of surgical enhancement of the lip that I use in my practice and involve autografts to the lips. The first is fat, which is harvested usually from the lower abdomen or medial thighs. The fat is centrifuged and placed into 1-mL syringes. A #3 Coleman cannula is used to place the fat in a similar technique to that used for the placement of filler. The vermilion border is enhanced first, followed by volumizing of the lip by placing product in the tubercles, making sure to create gentle mounds in these regions and then eversion, which is created by placing fat submucosally posterior to the wet/dry border of the lips.[11] The second surgical augmentation method for the lips involves the use of a SMAS harvested during a facelift. The length of each lip is measured and the appropriate length of the SMAS is harvested from each side of the face. The SMAS is appropriately contoured, being careful to evenly remove fat to provide a symmetric, smooth implant. An incision is made at just outside the oral commissure with an 11-blade. Curved Par scissors are used to create a submucosal pocket inside the vermilion border. A delicate liposuction cannula is placed through the incision and is used to form a space between the vermillion and the orbicularis oris by passing the cannula to an incision made on the opposite commissure. A tendon passer or alligator forceps is placed into the pocket entering one commissure and extending to the opposite commissure. The SMAS graft is then grasped and gently pulled through the lip until it is visualized at both openings. The lip is then gently palpated and stretched, and any remaining SMAS graft extending outside of the incisions is gently trimmed. The incision is closed using a 5-0 fast-absorbing gut.

Question 4: What technique do you use to resurface lines around the lips or perioral area?

DeJoseph

I prefer to resurface the lips using a fractional CO_2 laser. I find this technique blends moderate improvement with minimal complications and downtime for the patient. I anesthetize the perioral area with lidocaine blocks. Then the lips and entire perioral subunit from the melolabial (M/L) folds to the chin are resurfaced. My settings are a power or 20 W, density of 5 mm, and a duration of 3 ms. I routinely make 2 passes and occasional a third just on the vermillion. The laser I use is a Sandstome Matrix LS-25 for reference of settings. The area is dressed with Aquaphor for 4 to 5 days then a moisturizer afterward. I usually release patients for makeup in 1 week. Antiviral and antibacterial prophylaxis are always given starting 2 days prior. Patients are also counseled on sun avoidance for 1 month before and after the treatment to help prevent any pigmentation derangement.

That having been said, I have never seen any pigment issues with this technique in my practice.

AGARWAL

The most effective form of resurfacing in my hands has been fully ablative CO_2 laser resurfacing. For moderate to deeply ingrained rhytids, I counsel my patients to expect a 50% reduction in the depth of those rhytids with 1 session of fully ablative CO_2 resurfacing. Two to 3 passes using the Acupulse Superpulse CO_2 laser (Lumenis, Yokneam, Israel) are made in one session. Time to epithelialization is 10 to 14 days, with an ensuing 2 to 3 months of laser erythema. This laser treatment is used on individuals with Fitzpatrick skin type's I through III, using pretreatment and post-treatment hydroquinone and tretinoin cream for Fitzpatrick skin type III patients. It can be performed under local anesthetic infiltration in the office or with intravenous sedation in the operating room.

For those individuals with superficial to slightly moderate depth perioral rhytids, I recommend fractional CO_2 resurfacing for a 50% to 70% reduction in the depth of those rhytids. I use the Acupulse Fractional CO_2 laser (Lumenis) with the Acuscan120 Fractional Scanner. This allows for a combo mode in which deep fractional CO_2 laser energy is deposited first into the mid dermis, followed immediately by superficial fractional CO_2 laser energy into the epidermis. One pass is made, rarely followed by a second pass. Time to epithelialization is 8 to 10 days with an ensuing 6 weeks of laser erythema. Patients describe minimal to no pain after treatment with the fractional CO_2 laser, although there can be more bleeding and serous wound drainage after this treatment compared with the fully ablative CO_2 laser treatment.

Patient selection for each of these CO_2 laser modalities is of paramount importance. In my practice, superficial depth rhytids in Caucasian patients are always treated with fractional CO_2 laser resurfacing. To achieve optimal results for patients with moderate or deeply ingrained perioral rhytids, I recommend fully ablative CO_2 laser resurfacing. However, if a patient with moderate to severe perioral rhytids cannot afford the downtime associated with fully ablative CO_2 resurfacing, then I recommend fractional CO_2 laser resurfacing for a 30% reduction in the depth of those rhytids.

Finally, for those individuals with superficial perioral rhytids who cannot tolerate any downtime and are not interested in injectable treatments, I recommend a series of 4 Thermismooth radiofrequency treatments (ThermiGen, LLC, Irving, TX) performed by our aestheticians, with a subsequent single treatment performed every 6 months for maintenance. Temperature controlled radiofrequency heating of dermal collagen enables patients to achieve about a 30% reduction in the depth of their superficial vertical lip lines. Patients have been extremely pleased with this no downtime, yet effective treatment. Thermismooth treatments are not offered to those individuals with moderate to severe depth perioral rhytids because the patients will be uniformly disappointed.

GRECO

Resurfacing of the lips is accomplished with the Coherent Ultrapulse CO_2 laser. The deep perioral lines are marked with a blue surgical marking pen before surgery with the patient in a sitting position. The patient is asked to pucker intermittently to further define these lines. Each shoulder of a lip rhytid is then resurfaced with the finest computer programmed generated pattern, extending to the vermilion border if necessary for those rhytids responsible for lipstick bleed. This is performed with the use of ocular loops to better visualize the change in the laser tissue interactions. After the eschar is thoroughly removed, the entire perioral aesthetic unit is resurfaced as many times as necessary to improve the rhytids as much as possible. Resurfacing should cease when the skin turns a shammy color. Keep in mind a zone of necrosis will exist on a microscopic level that it will declare itself in the postoperative healing phase and result in further rhytid correction. With each pass of the laser, the diameter of the perioral area is marginally smaller to prevent an obvious line of demarcation in the perioral aesthetic unit. In addition, the last pass performed involves a low energy level of 250 mJ with a density of 4 in a triangular pattern to create an irregular outline of the periphery to distract the eye, similar to a running W-plasty used in scar revision. The decreasing diameters of each pass and the use of the triangular feathering pattern causes a subtle transitional change in the shade of the perioral region that is difficult to appreciate, even without makeup. If after 12 months of healing there remain a few lines, I offer dermabrasion with a wire brush, being careful to stabilize the lip by providing dental rolls underneath the lips for support. Only those persistent rhytids that have survived resurfacing are treated. These lines are usually found in patients who are active smokers. If a patient has had perioral resurfacing with CO_2 laser without significant improvement, the entire aesthetic unit is resurfaced using a wire brush dermabrasion with a diamond fraise dermabrasion at the periphery to feather the treatment area and prevent a line of demarcation between treated and untreated areas.

Question 5: What is your personal view on the aesthetic enhancement of the lips and recent trends you have observed?

DeJoseph

My personal view on lip enhancement is to maintain the natural lip architecture and size, not to create a "magazine photo shoot" size. Current preferences among patients vary significantly by generation. My more senior female patients want a subtle enhancement, mainly a platform for their lipstick and diminished vertical lines. My younger patients vary greatly from wanting a subtle change to a "wow-look-at-me" result. I do council all patients on the limitations of their expectations based on their natural lip build. I have refused patients in the past who want what I see as a ridiculous amount of volume, because they are my art work and represent my aesthetic also. Much of this desire in the younger patients stems from what is seen in modern celebrity pop culture. Full lips are in, as they say! Instagram and other social media platforms have captured their imagination like nothing else as they emulate their idols in wanting the lips like the fashion magazines. Again, I am not averse to this look, but it is on a patient-by-patient basis, according to their natural lip build. Some faces look great with really full lips, others do not. I always err on a lot of counseling regarding expectations and never straying from what I feel looks beautiful on a face. It has served me well thus far.

AGARWAL

There is no feature on the face that I have found to have more variation in terms of patients' ideal aesthetic shape and size than the lips. What is clear is that full lips are considered to be youthful and attractive. This belief has been confirmed in comparative studies between models and nonmodel controls, with the former group having greater upper and lower lip heights and lip angles as measured from the corners of the mouth.[12] I have found that most patients seeking lip augmentation for nonatrophic changes of the lips are between the ages of 18 and 25. This subset of patients often brings in photographs of popular icons in the fashion and music industry, many of whom have publicly highlighted their own lip augmentation procedures. The number one request has been to augment the upper lip more than the lower lip.

Second, lateral upper lip volume enhancement is a common request. Whereas I was originally taught during residency and fellowship that there should be more vermilion show of the lower lip compared with the upper lip, my view on this has changed, such that I now feel that the upper lip vermilion should be in 1:1 proportion with the lower lip vermilion. This gives a more sensual, balanced look. I also avoid accentuation of the white roll of the lip because I feel it gives an unnatural appearance.

A recent study in which images of attractive faces were digitally morphed to generate variations in upper to lower lip ratio, and then evaluated by a total of 428 conventional raters and Internet-based focused group raters, found a 1:2 ratio to be the most attractive.[13] However, my personal view when reviewing photographs presented in this study is that the 1:1 ratio is far more attractive than the 1:2 ratio. This finding highlights the nature of personal preference when it comes to evaluating lip aesthetics. My perception of beauty is far more consistent with the overwhelming majority of 1011 survey takers (60% of the 1011 respondents) who chose the 1.0:1.0 lip ratio as most attractive in a separate recent study.[14]

In addition to the trend toward a fuller upper lip, I have seen a decrease in the number of patients seeking surgical lip augmentation. This is in sharp contrast with a year-over-year increase in the number of nonsurgical lip injections that are performed. I believe the reversibility of lip injections offers peace of mind to patients, the lack of permanency gives them the opportunity to change their minds about lip fullness in the future, the cost of a syringe of filler performed twice a year is palatable to younger patients, and the fear of surgical manipulation of the lips in younger patients may all partially explain this trend.

GRECO

I view the lips as a pivotal aesthetic feature of the lower face, which possess incredible beauty when size and shape are aesthetically pleasing We have all seen those lips that when excessively volumized resemble 2 sausage links stacked on top of each other. The success of lip enhancement is found in maintaining the beautiful, delicate shape of the lips while providing enough volume, which gives them the attention they deserve as one of the key aesthetic features of the human face. Too much enhancement results in decimation of the delicate shape of the lips and can turn a patient's appearance into a caricature. A proper aesthetic enhancement of the lips creates a sense of sensuality that one finds endearing and captivating. Overenhancement destroys the delicate anatomy of the lips and results in the eyes roaming the face to find another oasis of aesthetic beauty.

It is also important to appreciate a person's dentition, as mentioned, when augmenting the lips. A class 2 or class 3 angles occlusion creates a challenge in providing balance on profile, as well as maintaining the appropriate proportion on anteroposterior view of the lips. Proper occlusion and aesthetic upper and lower dentition are important foundations to lip enhancement. Also related to occlusion is the shape and projection of the chin. The key to aesthetic enhancement of the lips is creating balance and symmetry while maintaining the delicate, beautiful anatomy that nature intended.

Question 6: How have your techniques in this area changed over the last 5 years?

DeJoseph

The main techniques I have changed over the years are surgical in nature. I no longer perform a vermillion advancement cheiloplasty for lip augmentation. I did this sparingly on some aging and very thin lips, and the results were good for the time. The aftermath of that procedure was complete loss of the white roll architecture and the need for makeup there constantly. I have abandoned this procedure as I and my patients became more sophisticated in our aesthetic for lips. Still, I had many satisfied patients, but it left me not feeling satisfied.

The other technique I no longer perform is commisureplasty. This technique was usually done in a severe aged face to turn the commissures up. It worked, but the scaring in my opinion was too obvious for more modern tastes. Now, I find I can achieve similar if not better results with filler to that area. Last, full ablative CO_2 laser resurfacing is something I no longer do. The results were modest at best, but the resultant late-term hypopigmentation was unacceptable to me. I found that, if patients were followed out long enough, almost all developed some level of perioral hyperpigmentation. This development required the use of makeup on a constant basis. I feel we have become much more savvy as surgeons and have better informed patients as to what good results are.

AGARWAL

The primary change in the last 5 years has been in my aesthetic view of the ideal proportion of the lips. I now feel that the 1:1 upper lip vermilion to lower lip vermilion ratio is most attractive for the majority of patients. I have also become more conservative when injecting filler in those individuals with extremely thin lips at baseline, because the degree of augmentation that can be achieved is limited, yet they can be rapidly tipped toward having overly prominent, protruding, unnatural appearing lips.

The other change has been in my treatment paradigm of aging patients with very early superficial fine upper lip rhytids, often accompanied by a slight reduction in upper lip volume. I offer 4 options to these patients depending on their goals. Treatment with onabotulinum toxin A (Allergan Inc.) or JUVEDERM Volbella XC can be used to treat superficial to moderate depth upper lip rhytids and achieve mild lip augmentation. Treatment of fine lines alone can be accomplished to a limited extent with Thermismooth radiofrequency treatments and more definitively with Acupulse Fractional CO_2 laser resurfacing.

I find that 5 to 6 units of onabotulinum toxin A injected in 4 injection sites is very useful in softening fine upper lip lines and slightly increasing upper lip vermilion show. My initial injection pattern several years ago included a fifth injection just above the vermilion border at the midline of the upper lip. However, this move created too much limitation of lip movement when patients would speak and also limited the use of a straw considerably. Since I eliminated the central upper lip injection site, and only inject at 4 injection sites (2 on each side of the upper lip lateral to the philtral columns and evenly spaced between the corners of the mouth and philtral columns), the incidence of upper lip restriction has been dramatically reduced. Patients are pleasantly surprised at how effective this simple treatment is.

From a surgical perspective, I have not had any significant modifications in the last 5 years. The limitations of volumization that can be achieved with nonsurgical or surgical lip augmentation in those patients with a long cutaneous upper lip have led me to recommend more subnasal lip lifts than I did previously. However, I have found that only a small fraction of patients choose to follow this recommendation.

GRECO

The technique of lip injection has changed primarily with the use of cannula over a needle. I have found that the cannula is much more gentle in the lip. The exact amount of material can be delivered in very accurate places without causing significant trauma. Because of the introduction of the cannula, I have found that my technique of injecting lips has changed to mirror the technique that I use when using structural fat grafting for lip enhancement. With the use of a 27-gauge, 1.5-inch cannula, I am able to provide augmentation to the vermillion border and I can also create a suitable augmentation to cupid's bow as well as to the philtral arches. The cannula is then directed into the wet/dry border portion of the lip and augmentation of the tubercles occurs. This is similar to what is done when structural fat grafting (SFG) is used to augment the lips. The last maneuver used in lip augmentation with a cannula is to evert the lip when passing the cannula posterior to the orbicularus oris muscle just submucosal in front of the frenulum of the upper and lower lip. A depot of filler is placed here and this will actually help with lip eversion. A similar technique is used with SFG; however, more linear threading and a greater volume of fat is used when creating the eversion to the lips by placing fat submucosally on the posterior aspect of the upper and lower lip.

REFERENCES

1. Farkas JP, Pessa JE, Hubbard B, et al. The science and theory behind facial aging. Plast Reconstr Surg Glob Open 2013;1(1):e8–15.
2. Klein AW. In search of the perfect lip: 2005. Dermatol Surg 2005;31:1599–603.
3. Jacono A. A new classification of lip zones to customize injectable lip augmentation. Arch Facial Plast Surg 2008;10(1):25–8.
4. Eccleston D, Murphy D. Juvederm® Volbella™ in the perioral area: a 12-month prospective, multicenter, open-label study. Clin Cosmet Investig Dermatol 2012;5:167–72.
5. Sarnoff D, Gotkin R. Six steps to the "perfect" lip. J Drugs Dermatol 2012;11(9):1081–8.
6. Moore KL. The developing human, clinical oriented embryology. In development of the face. Philadelphia: WB Saunders Company; 1982. p. 197–201.
7. Vartanian AJ, Frankel AS, Rubin MG. Injected hyaluronidase reduces restylane-mediated cutaneous augmentation. Arch Facial Plast Surg 2005;7(4):231–7.
8. Dayan SH, Arkins JP, Mathison CC. Management of impending necrosis associated with soft tissue filler injections. J Drugs Dermatol 2011;10(9):1007–12.
9. Agarwal A, Gracely E, Maloney R. Lip augmentation using sternocleidomastoid muscle and fascia grafts. Arch Facial Plast Surg 2010;12(2):97–102.
10. Raphael P, Harris R. Five-year experience with Perma Facial implant. Plast Reconstr Surg Glob Open 2014;2(5):1–9.
11. Coleman SR. Structural fat grafting. In aesthetic and anatomic considerations. St Louis (MI): Quality Medical Publishing, Inc; 2004. p. 204–35.
12. Bisson M, Grobbelaar A. The esthetic properties of lips: a comparison of models and nonmodels. Angle Orthod 2004;74(2):162–6.
13. Popenko N, Tripathi P, Devcic Z, et al. A quantitative approach to determining the ideal female lip aesthetic and its effect on facial attractiveness. JAMA Facial Plast Surg 2017;19(4):261–7.
14. Heidekrueger P, Juran S, Szpalski C, et al. The current preferred female lip ratio. J Craniomaxillofac Surg 2017;45(5):655–60.

Grafting Techniques in Primary and Revision Rhinoplasty

Brian J.F. Wong, MD, PhD[a,b,]*, Oren Friedman, MD[c],
Grant S. Hamilton III, MD[d]

KEYWORDS

- Rhinoplasty • Revision rhinoplasty • Costal cartilage • Auricular cartilage • Cartilage grafts

KEY POINTS

- Patient age, structural requirements, and airflow considerations are critical in selecting between septal, auricular, costal, and cadaveric cartilage tissue.
- There are many variants for spreader grafts placement and design.
- Remnant septal cartilage and auricular cartilage can be used in revision operations; consent for costal cartilage should be obtained, even if probability of rib graft harvest is low.
- Correction/augmentation of dorsal contour deformities are readily accomplished using monobloc and diced/shaved cartilage grafts. However, for airway expansion of the internal valve, dorsally extended spreaders should be considered.
- Tip grafting is nuanced and aesthetic objective must be balanced by considerations over available graft material and airway patency. Always consider turn in flaps and tip suture methods.

Panel discussion

1. How do you treat severe nasal valve collapse and a significant septal fracture deformity in an attractive patient who does not want any major changes in her appearance?

2. How would you manage a patient with a postseptoplasty dorsal depression who originally did not want any cosmetic changes to her nose?

3. How do you correct saddle deformities accompanied by a significant septal perforation?

4. Midvault surgery for obstruction and aesthetics can be challenging. What are considerations in the patient with a prominent dorsal hump? Also, how do you correct the convex lower lateral crura?

5. What grafting techniques can be used to contour and refine a bulbous nasal tip?

6. What grafting methods do you use to correct a pinched tip in secondary surgery?

7. What have you done differently over the past 5 years?

Disclosure: The authors have nothing to disclose.
[a] Division of Facial Plastic Surgery, Department of Otolaryngology–Head and Neck Surgery, University of California Irvine, 1002 Health Sciences Road, Irvine, CA 92617, USA; [b] Department of Biomedical Engineering, University of California Irvine, 1002 Health Sciences Road, Irvine, CA 92617, USA; [c] Facial Plastic Surgery, Department of Otorhinolaryngology–Head and Neck Surgery, University of Pennsylvania, 800 Walnut Street, 18th Floor, Philadelphia, PA 19107, USA; [d] Department of Otorhinolaryngology, Mayo Clinic, 200 First Street Southwest, Rochester, MN 55905, USA
* Corresponding author. Division of Facial Plastic Surgery, Department of Otolaryngology–Head and Neck Surgery, University of California Irvine, 1002 Health Sciences Road, Irvine, CA 92617.
E-mail address: bjwong@uci.edu

INTRODUCTION

Rhinoplasty has evolved immensely since the time of Joseph and has become more complex as both aesthetic standards and patient expectations have become more stringent. At the same time, despite improvements in surgical techniques guided by analysis of long-term outcomes, revision rates remain relatively low.[1-5] The cornerstone of contemporary rhinoplasty rests on structural cartilage grafting.[6] Structural grafts resist static forces owing to gravity and aging, and dynamic forces produced by tissue contraction, paranasal muscle activity, and oscillatory pressure gradients during respiration.[7-11] When properly performed, both airway patency and attractive contours are the anticipated surgical outcomes. Structural approaches in rhinoplasty remain dominant, and there has been a proliferation of graft use in both primary and secondary operations. Despite more than 100 years of progress, there is still no consensus about the best way to augment the dorsum, reshape and support the tip, or manage the middle third of the nose. Many controversies remain in rhinoplasty. This articles present different perspectives on these controversial topics.

In the dorsum, multiple approaches and techniques are used to correct deformities as subtle as a slight convexity and as dramatic as those seen in saddle noses affected by vasculitis. Options for correcting these defects, when extensive, can include a monobloc onlay graft, dorsally extended spreader grafts, camouflage grafts, and diced cartilage in fascia,[12] along with its many variants.[13] Septal, conchal, and costal cartilage can be used, with costal cartilage typically used for major deformities requiring strong structural support.

In the nasal tip, over the past decade, there has been a gradual shift away from the pro forma use of cap, shield, and columellar strut grafts and toward techniques that maintain native dome architecture and enhance mechanical stability.[14,15] Caudal septum extension grafts and their variants are now widely used to support the nasal tip, supplementing the popular classic floating columellar strut. Lower lateral cartilage malposition, crural convexity issues, and alar margin shape are treated with a number of techniques, including lateral crural strut grafts with or without repositioning. Less aggressive methods such as turn under flaps, mattress sutures, lateral crural tensioning,[16] and rim grafting,[17,18] are also used.

The middle vault is also a challenging area because it is an important part of the internal nasal valve and is responsible for a smooth brow-tip aesthetic line. Here, the spreader graft has remained the workhorse, although there are many different approaches beyond classic graft placement. Contemporary techniques include spreader flaps (auto spreader grafts),[19] as well as unique ways of reattaching separated upper lateral cartilage to the quadrangular cartilage.

The present article is not meant to be a comprehensive discourse on grafting, but focuses on a few illustrative case studies to demonstrate various techniques as well as controversies in graft placement and use to correct specific deformities.

Question 1: How do you treat severe nasal valve collapse and a significant septal fracture deformity in an attractive patient who does not want any major changes in her appearance?

Case 1: This healthy young woman has difficulty breathing at rest and during exercise (**Fig. 1A–D**). She has near total obstruction of the right nasal airway and no aesthetic concerns; her objective is to breathe better. On examination, with even a mild inspiratory effort, the left sidewall of her airway collapses. Intranasally, she has a severe septal fracture causing a deformity of the septum on the right side resulting in little airflow. This case is challenging in that the overall aesthetics of the patient are good and the patient is attractive. The septum is severely deformed, and this deformation extends to the dorsal quadrangular cartilage. There is also severe left spur and a deviation of the perpendicular plate to the right side, as expected.

FRIEDMAN

I always inquire about the patient's concerns as I try to address their specific needs and meet their expectations. In this case, the patient wishes to maintain her appearance but have improved breathing. My preference is to address the functional concerns and maintain the appearance just as the patient requested. The only way I can achieve this is through an endonasal approach, because if an external approach is used, I am unable to maintain an untouched tip and I will automatically be altering the shape of the nasal tip. I would apply a variety of techniques to straighten the septum, including resection of deviated portions of cartilage and bone, scoring the caudal septum and battening it with cartilage grafts, always maintaining a strong dorsal and caudal "L-strut." I would then add spreader grafts through an endonasal approach to stabilize the dorsal septum and improve the width of the nasal valve area. In this type of case, I also like to crush the inferior turbinates, as indicated, but I never remove

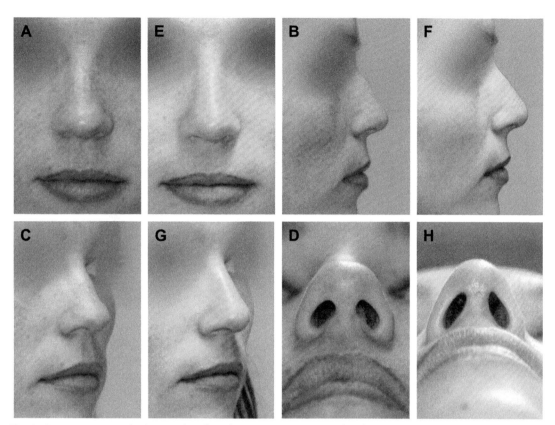

Fig. 1. Case 1, preoperative images (*A–D*) and postoperative images (*E–H*).

any tissue from the turbinates for fear of creating an iatrogenically induced atrophic rhinitis or empty nose syndrome. I like to apply Doyle splints in the nose in cases of significant septal deviations to ensure that the septum heals in the way I left it in the operating room. If I feel that she has weak external nasal valve support, I might also add an external valve batten graft, either through a small marginal incision or through an external alar–facial stab incision. The graft is placed in a precise pocket along the nostril rim to support the external valve either through a marginal incision (**Fig. 2**A) or through a stab incision in the alar–facial crease (**Fig. 2**B).[20]

HAMILTON

This patient, with no aesthetic concerns, needs a septoplasty and possibly some reinforcement of her lateral nasal wall. Although she collapses on the left with inspiration, this may be because her right side is completely obstructed. She is essentially breathing 2 nostrils of air through just the left side. This increases the velocity and, therefore, decreases the pressure of the air passing through her left nasal passage. Sometimes in patients like

this a septoplasty is all that is needed. However, she does have a rounded tip and may have some internal recurvature of her lateral crura. In that case, I would perform an endonasal septoplasty and harvest enough septal cartilage for 2 alar batten grafts. These grafts can also be placed endonasally through a marginal incision. I find that making a small 90° cut from the lateral aspect of the marginal incision toward the alar rim facilitates placement of the graft. Because I am placing the graft, I have a low threshold for excising the recurvate part of the lateral crus and replacing it with the flat batten. I place the graft obliquely to the long axis of the lateral crus to better reinforce the area of supra-alar pinching. It does not extend toward the lateral canthus like the lateral crus. Instead, it is oriented more in the direction of the ear lobule. In addition, I place bolsters on the sidewalls of the nose whenever I operate on the external nasal valve. I find that this helps to prevent migration of the grafts and minimizes edema formation and possible medialization of the lateral nasal wall.

When the caudal septum is crooked, it is often due to one (or two) of two types of problems. Sometimes the caudal septum is inherently curved or cupped. In these cases I often excise the caudal

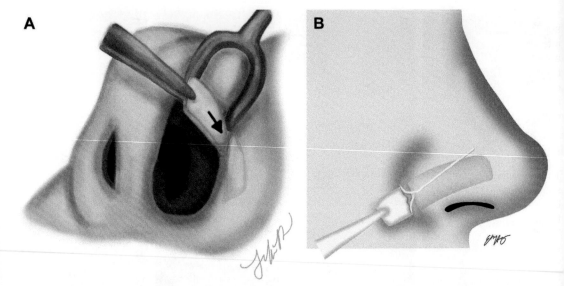

Fig. 2. External valve batten grafts placed via marginal incision (*A*) and via external alar crease incision (*B*). (*Courtesy of* Ellen Hong, BS, University of California Irvine, Irvine, CA.)

septum and replace it with a straight piece from the posterior quadrangular cartilage. In other cases, the caudal septum is fairly straight but is displaced from the midline. When this happens, I reposition the caudal septum and may reinforce it with a septal batten graft. I typically outfracture the inferior turbinates and occasionally I reduce them with a submucous resection. I also like to use Doyle splints. I find them effective at preventing hematoma formation and adding some support to the septum in the immediate postoperative period in the event of an inadvertent bump to the nose.

WONG

The open approach was selected to obtain panoramic access to the septum, which was fairly tortuous especially caudally. A left-sided maxillary crest spur was reduced and the perpendicular plate was thinned using an ultrasonic debrider (Sonopet, Stryker, Kalamazoo, MI). Next, the off-center posterior septal angle was disarticulated and reattached to the nasal spine in the midline. Symmetric spreader grafts were placed to straighten the dorsal quadrangular cartilage and widen the internal nasal valve (**Fig. 1**E). I did soften the microhump using the sonopet as I often loose 0.25 to 0.55 mm of dorsal height when separating upper laterals from the septum (**Fig. 1**F, G). Tip support was reestablished with a boomerang septal extension graft that embraced the anterior septal angle in an end-to-end fashion (**Fig. 3**). A single suture incorporating the extension graft, and both domes reestablished the nasal tip.

Medial crura were attached to the extension graft as well. The key issue here is that the septal extension graft specifies every aspect of the lateral profile. Tip bifidity is reestablished by careful and measured placement of the extension graft–domal sutures; there was a very minimal reduction in bifidity (**Fig. 1**H), but the overall change is extremely subtle.

Question 2: How would you manage a patient with a postseptoplasty dorsal depression who originally did not want any cosmetic changes to her nose?

Case 2: This patient had surgery (performed elsewhere) to correct nasal obstruction. Before that operation, she had no aesthetic concerns

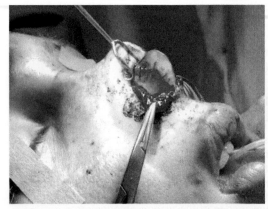

Fig. 3. "Boomerang" septal extension graft placed end to end with anterior septal angle and secured with multiple "figure-of-8" sutures.

about her nose (**Fig. 4**A–D). She had undergone a septoplasty, right concha bullosa, and bilateral inferior turbinate reductions. After that initial operation, she noticed that the shape of her nose began to change. She also had persistent nasal obstruction. She has medium thickness skin, a noticeable saddle nose, some right external valve collapse, and a left caudal septal deviation.

FRIEDMAN

This young and attractive female patient has a saddle nose deformity, an associated broad and boxy nasal tip, and an overrotated nose. All of these elements are likely the result of loss of at least the dorsal septum support, but very possibly even more septal support. As with every patient, I would like to assess what their expectations are of the surgery and then determine if I could help the patient achieve those goals. Second, I would need to understand what the intranasal examination looks like to determine what her surgery might entail. If there is inadequate septal cartilage available, I might proceed with ear cartilage reconstruction. However, if the skin is tightly adherent to the underlying nasal skeleton, and if there is an insufficient amount of native septal cartilage, I would not hesitate to proceed with autologous rib graft harvest.

My preferred method for reconstruction of this patient's nose would include an external approach, followed by bony dorsal rasping to reduce the bony deformity and create a smoother and lower profile bony dorsum. This step would be followed by the application of bilateral spreader grafts to help support the weakened/lost dorsal septum support that is causing the saddling and rotation and boxy tip changes. The spreaders would stand taller (dorsally extended) than the current nasal dorsum to align the cartilaginous dorsum with the bony dorsal height. The upper lateral cartilages that were released from the dorsal septum would then be unfurled and stretched to reach the new dorsal height, and they would be secured to the newly stabilized and elevated dorsum. If additional dorsal height was required, a cartilage onlay graft could be applied, and finally, a smoothening layer of fascia or manipulated cartilage would be applied. The overly rotated and widened tip would be addressed with transdomal and interdomal sutures, possibly a small cephalic trim with or without a turn-in flap for added

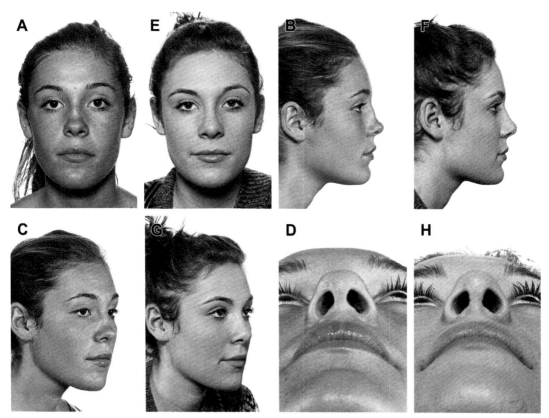

Fig. 4. Case 2, preoperative images (A–D) and postoperative images (E–H).

strength and flattening of the widened tip carti-lages. The spreader grafts that recreated dorsal support would also be used to push the tip down-ward to derotate the tip of the nose. The middle and medial crura would be secured to the extended spreader grafts to lengthen and derotate the nasal tip, and a columellar strut or septal extension graft might be required if the native caudal septum was weak. The decision to use auricular or costal cartilage would be made based on the amount of skin contracture present be-tween the skin and underlying skeleton at present, but in most likelihood, I would use rib grafts to sup-port the next construct of this patient's nose, given the anticipated wound contracture and her young age.

WONG

There are numerous techniques that can be used to treat a dorsal concavity. This is an attractive patient who has a saddle, and a previous septoplasty oper-ation. One would assume this is iatrogenic, although in theory she may have some sort of auto-immune process like Wegener's granulomatosis,

which could easily be eliminated as a cause by ordering a cytoplasmic antineutrophil cytoplasmic antibody test.[21] Assuming that there are no medical contraindications to surgery and that this deformity is long-standing, meaning stable for more than 1 year, one could consider surgical correction. There are a lot of options here, including monobloc augmentation (method illustrated in **Fig. 5**), dorsally extended spreaders (method illustrated in **Fig. 6**), diced cartilage in fascia and its variants including Tasman type techniques, and even in the appro-priate patient injections using fillers.[22–24]

My decisions are largely based on the airway, in that correction of the contour alone may not in-crease airspace within the midvault. It may not be necessary in this patient, but for the sake of argument let's assume that there is some element of nasal airway obstruction in the midvault. If that is the case, and there is no septal perforation, I would harvest costal cartilage via a very small inframammary incision, precisely section the carti-lage[25] creating rather long slender strips (1.5 mm or 2.0 mm in thickness; **Fig. 7**A), which I would extend dorsally to correct the contour. In general, using a guillotine slicer, I can readily obtain up to

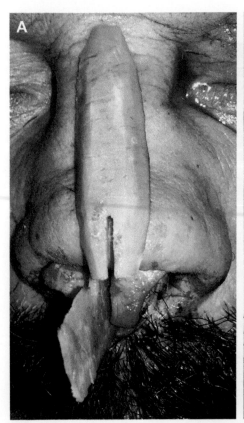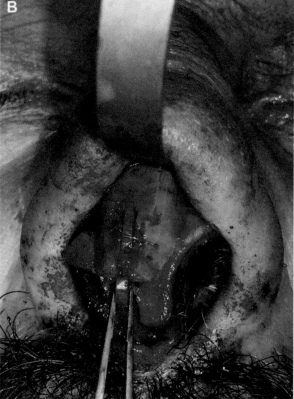

Fig. 5. Dorsal augmentation using mono block cartilage graft, notched at the end (A) and secured to caudal septal extension graft with dovetailed carving (B).

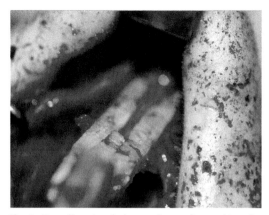

Fig. 6. Dorsally extended spreader grafts used to raise the midvault height.

5 fairly uniform cartilage specimens from 1 rib, which provides plenty of very uniform cartilage specimens (**Fig. 7**B) for reconstruction even in partially calcified specimens (**Fig. 7**C). If the native dorsal septum cannot support these extended spreaders or if the skin soft tissue envelope is too retracted, then I would add support with the

septal extension graft using costal cartilage cut to 1.0 mm in thickness. This would be a bit of a challenge in a young patient because it is more difficult it is to predict the degree of curvature even when sectioning tissue using Gillies and Gibson's balanced cross-sections.[26,27] The technical challenge here is making sure that the transition between the cephalic terminus of the spreader grafts is in line with what looks like overall to be a reasonably positioned distal nasal bone terminus.

Bringing the upper lateral cartilages back up to meet these extended spreader grafts can be a challenge. Relaxing incisions running parallel to the long axis of the nose that are partial thickness through the perichondrium facilities some stretch of the septal mucoperichondrium, I have been able to get up to 7 mm of stretch on 1 occasion. Here she does not need that much and I think it would be unnecessary to make these relaxing incision that are akin to galeotomies in the scalp.

Again, the rationale for using extended spreader grafts is because you expand the midvault cross-sectional area, and correct abnormalities of the internal nasal valve. In the absence of obstruction, any onlay technique would serve this patient well

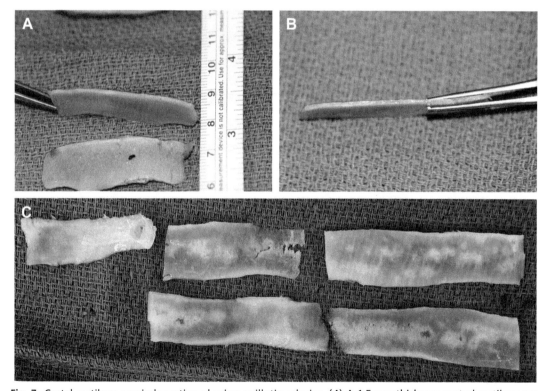

Fig. 7. Costal cartilage precisely sectioned using guillotine device. (*A*) A 1.5-mm thickness central cartilage sections, (*B*) edge on view of graft, and (*C*) five 1.5-mm-thick grafts harvested from one costal cartilage graft in partially calcified section (scale bar 1 cm).

also. It is challenging because she has 70 years ahead of her, and most of these techniques with the exception of the placement of the monobloc cartilage, are still relatively new with less than 40 years of long-term experience.

HAMILTON

I harvested some costal cartilage because her septum lacked cartilage that could have potentially useful for grafting. After exposing her septum, it became apparent that her saddle was a consequence of inadequate structural support of her dorsal septal strut. To reinforce this, I placed spreader grafts to act as a foundation for a solid dorsal graft. I also reinforced her caudal septum with a thin piece of cartilage as a septal batten. From the costal cartilage, I made a solid dorsal graft. Before placing it, I reduced her nasal bones enough to make room for the cartilage, because I did not want to raise her bony dorsum. I also placed alar batten grafts to help with her external nasal valve collapse. Finally, I placed a shield graft with some perichondrium at the tip for camouflage. These photos show her 1 year postoperative result (**Fig. 4**E–H).

Question 3: How do you correct saddle deformities accompanied by a significant septal perforation?

Case 3: This patient is a 55-year-old man who had a malignant sinonasal mass excised with resultant septal perforation and associated saddle nose deformity and columellar retraction (**Fig. 8**A–D). He had a widened dorsum associated with the saddle deformity as well as functional compromised owing to sidewall collapse.

HAMILTON

This man has an obvious loss of support in the lower two-thirds of his nose resulting in a saddle nose deformity, widened front view, and an acute nasolabial angle. Common options for reconstructing a saddle nose include placing a dorsal onlay graft made of solid or diced cartilage. Less commonly, spreader grafts can be placed that extend above the dorsal septum to provide the appropriate amount of dorsal projection. These patients often have a deficiency of dorsal septum owing to a septal perforation or overzealous cartilage excision during a septoplasty.

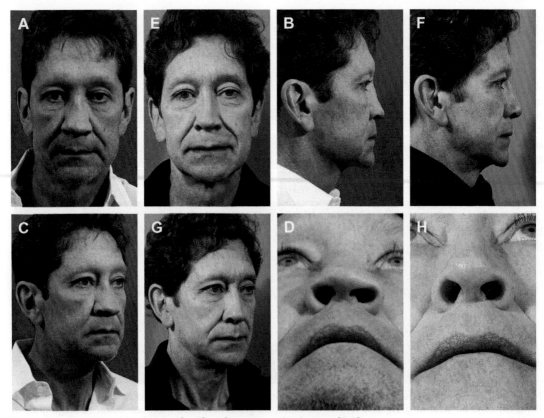

Fig. 8. Case 3, preoperative images (*A–D*) and postoperative images (*E–H*).

Under such circumstances it can be very challenging to place spreader grafts because there is not much existing dorsal structure to which the grafts can be affixed. Placing only tall spreader grafts or an onlay of solid or diced cartilage will only solve a part of this man's problem. In addition to dorsal augmentation, he needs support of his nasal base. His nostrils have become flared and horizontally oriented owing to deprojection of his tip. Base support can be accomplished with a caudal extension graft and fixation of the medial crura to it. In my opinion, a floating columellar strut is unlikely to provide enough projection and certainly will not improve the contour of the nasolabial angle.

My preference for dorsal augmentation is a solid autologous costal cartilage graft. I like this solution for 2 reasons. First, I know that the graft is going to be smooth. Second, I can integrate a solid dorsal graft with a caudal extension or caudal replacement graft to reconstitute a structurally sound L-strut. In this man, I would harvest enough costal cartilage for a dorsal and caudal support. In most cases this is about 6 cm. In addition to the cartilage, I would remove a strip of perichondrium to be used for softening the edges of cartilage grafts, filling in small defects and helping the dorsal graft adhere to the nasal bones.

It is often necessary to remove some of the bony dorsum to make room for the dorsal graft, even in patients without a dorsal hump. Sewing a small piece of perichondrium to the undersurface of the caudal end of the dorsal graft will help it to adhere to the bones. Patients like this are often missing the caudal septum, resulting in poor tip support, a long upper lip, and an acute nasolabial angle. Replacing the caudal septum and affixing the medial crura to it can support the base of the nose, improve projection, reposition a retracted columella, and restore a natural nasal contour. It is necessary when using a solid dorsal graft to create a stable joint between the caudal and dorsal grafts. I typically make a small tongue-in-groove joint that is easily modified to set an appropriate amount of tip projection. I place a suture or two through the joint to help with stability in the immediate postoperative period.

WONG

This is a challenging case. He has loss of dorsal height, and may have some element of airway compromise. Potentially, any of the methods Dr Hamilton mentions will work well to achieve a good cosmetic outcome. One concern when using any form of onlay graft alone to raise dorsal height is that airway obstruction may not improve. L-strut reconstruction using a dorsal onlay and caudal septal replacement alone may not adequately increase the cross-sectional airway through the gateway region (internal nasal valve) of the nose.[28] I prefer to raise the internal height of the airway through the gateway region of the nose. For this case, rib would be the only option for me, because the degree of dorsal augmentation required is substantial. This patient has a second issue in that the radix is a bit lower than I prefer, and I would like to reposition his starting point more cephalically to give a bit more strength and masculinity to his appearance. My approach would be open, and I would harvest rib and perichondrium. I would need at least 4 cm of rib, and would section it precisely into multiple segments 1.5 or 2.0 mm in thickness (see **Fig. 7**). The straightest central segment would be used as a septal replacement or extension graft, and I would secure it to the nasal spine or existing caudal septum (side to side). The upper lateral cartilages would be separated from the septum. An extended spreader graft would be used here and it would need to span the distance from the septal extension graft to the new radix point. Dorsally, it would be extended to raise the dorsum (see **Fig. 6**). The use of a dorsally extended or "proud" spreader is key to establishing the correct lateral profile. This reconstructs the L-strut much in the manner Dr Hamilton described, but also expands the cross-sectional airway area. There are 3 challenging issues with this approach. First, the rib needs to be sectioned precisely, and the technical details of this approach are discussed elsewhere.[25] Second, the upper lateral cartilage complex would have to be "stretched" to reach the neodorsum for reattachment, as discussed in the second case. A septal perforation would be a relative contraindication to using this approach, and it depends on the size of the perforation, which, if small, could be repaired at the same time. Finally, when extending a spreader graft cephalically, it may be notched (**Fig. 9**) to articulate with the caudal terminus of the nasal bones centrally; this also provides stability and can more cephalically position the radix like a radix graft. Once placed and secured (sutured to dorsal septum), it is trimmed and contoured to establish the desired profile. The overlapping of extended spreader and nasal bone can lead to irregularities in the dorsum, so cartilage "scales" are placed to smooth this transition.[29] Rib perichondrium, which is rather thick, is placed over the entire spreader graft, upper

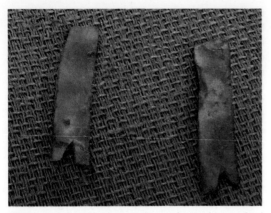

Fig. 9. Costal cartilage spreader grafts can be notched cephalically, and designed to articulate with the caudal aspect of the nasal bones. They are then secured to the dorsal quadrangular cartilage. They are trimmed and contoured to establish the desired lateral profile. Scale bar 1 cm.

lateral complex. The tip would be reconstructed as Dr Hamilton specified.

FRIEDMAN

He underwent auricular cartilage harvest, because there was inadequate septal cartilage available. In addition, temporalis fascia was harvested and a diced cartilage fascia graft was fashioned. Ear cartilage was diced to 1- to 2-mm cubes. The temporalis fascia was wrapped around a 1-mL syringe and the diced cartilage was inserted into the tubed temporalis fascia. The diced cartilage fascia graft was then placed endonasally along the dorsum of the nose to correct the saddle deformity. An additional diced cartilage fascia graft was placed through a hemitransfixion incision along the premaxillary region to project the tip by providing improved columellar support. A columellar strut graft was applied to help maintain tip projection. In this fashion, we provided added dorsal support through an onlay graft and projected the tip to enhance the aesthetics and function in a minimally invasive fashion (**Fig. 8**E–H).

Question 4: Midvault surgery for obstruction and aesthetics can be challenging. What are considerations in the patient with a prominent dorsal hump? Also, how do you correct the convex lower lateral crura?

Case 4: This 45-year-old woman presents for improvement in both nasal appearance and breathing (see **Fig. 12**A–D). She is not satisfied with the dorsal prominence, the ptotic tip, and the visible crease between the medial crura at the tip. She is 5 feet 8 inches tall and wants a "natural appearing, nonoperated looking nose."

HAMILTON

This woman has a small dorsal hump and a pollybeak that I suspect is due to a prominent anterior septal angle. In addition, she looks to be slightly underrotated and overprojected. She seems to have medium-thin skin and a divergence of her domes and supratip, resulting in a depression in her tip. When removing a dorsal hump, the upper lateral cartilages are often separated from the dorsal septum. In patients like this, there are several options for managing the middle third of the nose. Spreader grafts are probably the most commonly used method for preventing collapse of the internal nasal valve. I almost always use spreader grafts, but I have started using them in a slightly different way than what is typically described. The usual way to place a spreader graft through the external approach is to sew a strip of cartilage (the graft) between the septum and the upper lateral cartilage. What I do is to remove the dorsal hump by excising only the dorsal septum, leaving the upper lateral cartilages unmodified. This results in a relative excess of upper lateral cartilage that can be used advantageously. After separating the upper lateral cartilages from the septum and excising the excess dorsum, I make 2 spreader grafts and sew them to the septum 1 to 2 mm below the dorsal edge of the septum (**Fig. 10**). This maneuver allows me enough room to attach the upper lateral cartilages to the septum in an end-to-side manner. I think this has several advantages. First, the upper lateral cartilages are cantilevered outward by the spreader graft instead of being laterally displaced. Second, I find it easier to get a smooth contour to the lateral aspect of the dorsum because the upper lateral cartilages are returned to a position that is closer to their natural anatomic one. In effect, this mimics the effect of an endonasally placed spreader graft but through the open approach, although here the spreader graft functions as a stud both resisting downward forces and cantilevering the upper lateral cartilage upward.

This patient also has slightly convex lateral crura. If she wants to correct her rounded tip, my preferred method is to place lateral crural strut grafts by first creating a precise pocket beneath the lower ala (**Fig. 11**A) and then inserting the graft into position (**Fig. 11**B). Lateral crural strut grafts are flat, thin, elastic strips of cartilage placed between the lateral crus and vestibular skin. If I am using rib, especially in an older patient with more brittle cartilage, I use the peripheral layer of cartilage because it can be shaved quite thin while still being strong and elastic enough to resist cracking. Beside reshaping the convex lateral crura, strut

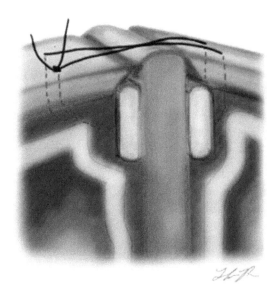

Fig. 10. Cantilevered upper lateral cartilages rest on spreader grafts placed 1 to 2 mm beneath the quadrangular cartilage contour. Attaching an upper lateral cartilage in this manner expands the valve region and aids in establishing a smooth dorsum. (*Courtesy of Tiffany Pham, BS, University of California Irvine, Irvine, CA.*)

grafts can also support the lateral nasal wall and improve the patency of the external nasal valve. In patients who have very convex lateral crura, there can be some unintended tip projection and counterrotation as the curved lateral crura are flattened and become longer. In these cases, dividing and overlapping the lateral crura several millimeters lateral to the dome can counteract both the projection and counterrotation.

WONG

The approach to the midvault that Dr Hamilton advocates is intriguing and structurally makes quite a bit of sense. With regard to the nasal tip, correcting the convexity of the tip can be accomplished a number of ways. Given that she has cartilaginous support through her soft triangle facet, and along the alar margin, almost any technique will work, from a simple dome suture to lateral crural division to strut grafts. I prefer to perform a lateral crural tensioning maneuver[30] combined with an end-to-end caudal extension graft (see **Fig. 3**), in this particular case (see case 6). My rationale is that this requires very little cartilage use, and is a conservative noncartilage splitting procedure. I think that in this patient strut grafts will work well, but could be a problem in patients with narrow nasal inlets.

FRIEDMAN

I performed an external rhinoplasty to address the poorly defined tip with a crease between the medial crura and ptosis. To reduce the dorsum, I separated the upper lateral cartilages from the dorsal septum, reduced the cartilaginous dorsum, and then turned in the upper lateral cartilages to serve as turn-in autospreader flaps.[31] I was concerned about visible irregularities through her thin skin and the turn-in flap provided a nice option for the smoothest dorsal contour. The turn in flaps were secured to the dorsal septum with 5-0 PDS suture. The tip was then treated with transdomal and interdomal sutures to (1) contour and support, (2) deproject, and (3) narrow the tip. In addition, crushed septal cartilage was placed between the domes to soften the visible crease between the medial crura, which was the patient's greatest preoperative complaint. The patient experienced improvements in both breathing and appearance with this technique (**Fig. 12E–H**).

Question 5: What grafting techniques can be used to contour and refine a bulbous nasal tip?

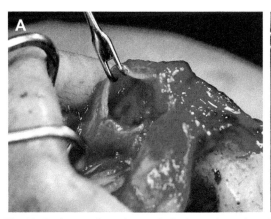
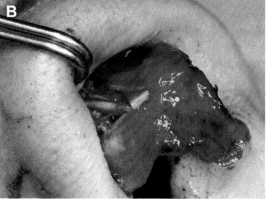

Fig. 11. Pocket made underneath the lower lateral cartilage (*A*) to accommodate a lateral crural strut graft, and (*B*) graft inserted into position.

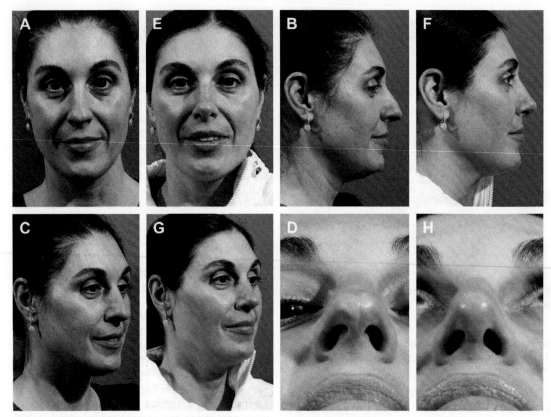

Fig. 12. Case 4, preoperative images (*A–D*) and postoperative images (*E–H*).

Case 5: This patient had both breathing and aesthetic concerns. Her nasal obstruction was multifactorial because she had environmental allergies and a significant septal deviation (**Fig. 13**A–D). On examination of her nose, I found her septum badly deviated to the right and a right-sided concha bullosa. She also had medium thickness skin and a small chin.

WONG

This is an interesting case that is notable for a nose that has a slight dorsal convexity, combined with a rather amorphous nasal tip, and a somewhat indistinct infratip lobule. I will skip the details with respect to the midvault and dorsum because this is a tip problem. What is telling from the base view is that she does not have any issue with respect to crowding of external valve airspace. This opens up a number of possibilities for treatment. With respect to correcting the curvature or convexity of the lateral crura, there are a number of techniques that can be used here. She does not have malposition of lateral crura and she seems to have good stability across the alar margin and soft triangle.

In my hands, I get the most consistent outcomes approaching this open, and I do think that there is

a very small hump that could be corrected first of all. The septum would be addressed via this anterior approach, avoiding Killian or Cottle incisions. The septal deformity would be corrected, and cartilage would be harvested for graft placement. My priority is the flattest and straightest cartilage tissue is reserved for septal extension grafts and articulated rim grafts. In individuals of European ancestry, I generally have adequate cartilage in primary cases. With other ethnicities, I generally consent for conchal cartilage, as a precaution. The least uniform cartilage tissue from the septum I reserve for spreader grafts, which I would place in this patient.

I would address the convexity using a combination of a septal extension graft combined with a lateral crural tensioning maneuver.[16,30] The septal extension graft would be critical in my approach to the nasal tip because it provides an anchor point to attach the new domes and still maintain to some degree rigid fixation. I would place the septal extension graft end to end using a "boomerang" type configuration (see **Fig. 3**), which embraces the anterior septal angle. I secure these using a series of interrupted figure-of-8 sutures, although occasionally I add very thin cartilage buttressed grafts in this area. The

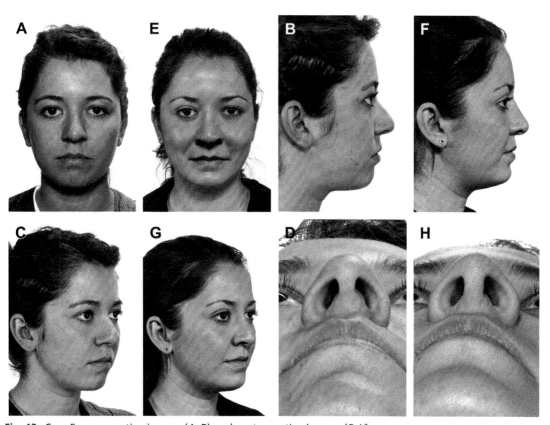

Fig. 13. Case 5, preoperative images (*A–D*) and postoperative images (*E–H*).

septal extension graft lets me very accurately set the tip defining point, the supratip breakpoint. The shape of her alar lobule is just as critical to me, because I do not like her lateral profile. She could benefit from more rotation, but I think it is more in this case of lacking a distinct infratip breakpoint. Often, however, with lateral crural tensioning, you do expose or create weakness in the lateral alar lobule, at which point I would place an articulated alar rim graft. This would stabilize the alar margin, strengthen the soft triangle facet, soften an alar margin furrow, and protect against potential parenthesis sign deformations. Articulate alar rim grafts are of exceptional value when the external nasal valve airspace is limited (thin narrow nasal space).[17,18]

FRIEDMAN

This patient has a dorsal convexity, significantly low radix with the deepest point of the radix located at the pupil, a beautifully triangulated and symmetric tip on base view with an open external nasal valve, and a very broad nasal tip on frontal view likely owing to slight cephalic malposition of the lower lateral cartilage or simply excessive height of the lateral crura with an otherwise

relatively smooth brow-tip aesthetic line. There is slight asymmetry to the lateral crura in terms of width, but not too dramatic. There is a slightly acute nasolabial angle with a weak columella relative to the ala, which is most pronounced at the base of the columella. There are many ways to address these issues, and much of the decision on how to approach the nose would stem from my discussion with the patient. First and foremost, I would like to know what the patient wants to achieve from the surgery, and with that I would establish how I could best satisfy her stated goals. My general philosophy is to do as little as necessary to achieve the patient's goals, and in this patient's case, that would most likely be achieved through an endonasal approach.

Generally speaking, I believe the patient's dorsal line would benefit from a combination of lowering the cartilaginous dorsum and raising the radix with a cartilaginous radix graft. I would aim to create a tip–supratip differential of 1 to 2 mm, which I think could be established primarily through a reduction of the cartilaginous dorsum, but could be augmented as necessary with a camouflaging tip graft made of bruised cartilage. Slight rotation of the tip and narrowing of the excessively full tip would be established with a minimal cephalic trim in combination with the cartilaginous dorsal reduction that would add to the appearance of rotation. The nasolabial angle is acute and due to a weakness at the base of the columella, giving the sense of less rotation than there actually is, so I might add a columellar strut/plumping graft to create more of an obtuse angle and a better alar–columellar relationship. I expect this to also strengthen the tip support to insure the tip–supratip differential is achieved and maintained. Spreader grafts would stabilize the middle third, given the dorsal reduction and potential weakening of middle third support created by the dorsal reduction. Radix graft would be achieved with an onlay camouflage graft of slightly bruised cartilage, possibly secured with transcutaneous sutures that are Steri-Stripped to the skin before application of the external cast.

HAMILTON

During surgery, I began with a chin implant placed through a submental incision. After turning my attention to her nose, I used an open approach to place spreader grafts, a radix graft (**Fig. 14**), and batten grafts in the form of lateral crural strut grafts. I placed them by making a small cephalic trim and dissecting a pocket between the lateral crus and the vestibular skin. I make the pocket oblique to the long axis of the lateral crus to provide more support to the lateral nasal wall. These strut grafts were placed primarily to reshape her rounded tip, although they also provide reinforcement to the external nasal valve. They did cause a little flaring of her nostrils, so I also performed a conservative alar base reduction. For tip support, I placed a columellar strut. The postoperative result shown is from 4 years after surgery (**Fig. 13**E–H).

Question 6: What grafting methods do you use to correct a pinched tip in secondary surgery?

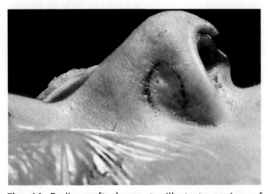

Fig. 14. Radix graft shown to illustrate region of placement.

Case 6: This healthy young woman had 2 cosmetic rhinoplasty operations performed elsewhere, and was unhappy with the "sausage nose" appearance of her tip, as well as the inability to breath with moderate inspiratory efforts (**Fig. 15**A–D). Originally, a "hump" reduction was performed in the first operation, followed by a second procedure aimed at correcting her septum. She believes the hump is improved but does not like her tip. She cannot breathe. The previous surgeon's operative reports provided little detail, and it is vague with respect to whether septal cartilage was removed. Her examination was notable for very narrow internal nasal valve angles, a posterior septal angle disarticulated off the nasal spine. There is a Cottle incision scar, residual septal spurs, and on cotton tip applicator palpation, no clear submucous resection defect. The dorsum is slightly irregular to touch.

HAMILTON

This young woman has a challenging problem. First, she seems to have thin skin based on her freckles. Her breathing problems are at least partly a result of having a very narrow nose and narrow nostrils. She also has some supra-alar pinching and collapse of her external valves with inspiration. In addition, her tip looks to be a little overprojected, which is exacerbated by her overreduced dorsum. To address these problems, it will likely be necessary to harvest some rib cartilage. During the preparatory part of the operation, I would palpate her septum while injecting it to assess for the presence of any remaining cartilage. I would use an open approach and expose her nasal skeleton. I would deproject her tip and set her medial crura back onto a caudal extension graft. I would also make an elongated radix graft that would taper to approximately the rhinion to further decrease the appearance of her overprojection. Her lateral crura present the greatest challenge of this operation. I think they are too sagittally malpositioned in that the short axes of the lateral crura are likely nearly parallel to the septum. This would explain her narrow nostrils and the "ball-like" appearance of her tip. By elevating the caudal margins of the lateral crura, she would have more of an arch to her base view instead of the alar pinching that she had preoperatively. This reorientation would also open her external nasal valves and improve her breathing. I would do this with a combination of lateral crural strut grafts and repositioning sutures. With her thin skin, it would be necessary to camouflage the cartilages in her tip to prevent them from showing as the edema resolves.

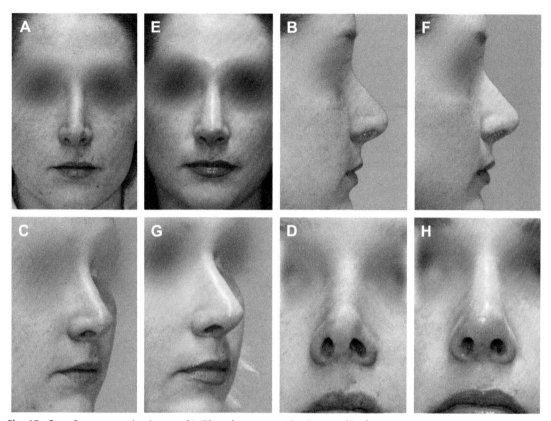

Fig. 15. Case 6, preoperative images (*A–D*) and postoperative images (*E–H*).

FRIEDMAN

This is a young female patient with thin skin and significant asymmetry of the lower third of the nose and supra-alar pinching. She demonstrates static and dynamic collapse of the nasal sidewall causing significant airway obstruction. Overall the brow-tip aesthetic line looks nice on resting frontal view, the profile view looks reasonable, and the area that requires the greatest work, in my mind, is the nasal tip. To create the better symmetry at the tip I would need to approach this patient through an external rhinoplasty to release all of the contracted skin and then create a stronger, more symmetric skeletal support at the tip that would hopefully withstand the contractile forces of wound healing. She would require a septal extension graft, either end to end or side to side, as well as rim grafts secured to the medial crura to create a more symmetric relationship at the dome and between the right and left ala. Attention would be paid to correcting the asymmetry between the right and left ala–columellar relationships. Spreader grafts would be used to maintain the midline dorsum in a straight position; it seems to be slightly crooked on inspiratory frontal view. Based on

the prior surgeries, the patient would likely need cartilage harvested from other sources, whether this would be autologous rib or ear would depend on how much, if any, native nasal cartilage is available for use, or if any of the previous surgeries' cartilage could be recycled and reused.

WONG

This was a very reasonable patient who had expectations of nasal tip improvement and airway patency. I had obtained consent for both conchal and costal cartilage, although on examination I did not feel a distinct SMR defect. The open approach was used, and an anterior approach to the septum quickly identified largely intact septal cartilage. Fortunately, there was only a small SMR defect at the junction of the perpendicular plate, vomer, and quadrangular cartilage. There was a residual deformation of the perpendicular plate. Upper lateral cartilages were not attached to the dorsal septum. Alar cartilages were asymmetric and a single 3-0 nylon type suture was identified at the posterior septal angle. Cartilage was harvested from the remaining septum. The perpendicular plate along with a deviation of the dorsal septum were responsible for the airway obstruction. Rather than resect or simply displace the perpendicular plate with gentle pressure, I use a septal burr (Medtronic, Minneapolis, MN) or ultrasonic device to contour and thin the plate first, then displace it gently to open up the airway. A PDS foil (0.15 mm thickness, perforated) was fashioned in the shape of the L-strut and used as a "tension–compression" band to further straightening the dorsum.[32,33] To accomplish this, numerous PDS sutures are placed to create a proper balance of forces.

Conventional spreader grafts and an end-to-end "boomerang" septal extension graft were then secured. For the tip, lateral crural tensioning was performed (**Fig. 16**) with recruitment of 4 mm of crura. This was followed by a paradomal cephalic trim (1 × 4 mm of tissue removed), and placement of articulated alar rim grafts (20 × 5 mm, right triangular in shape). The tensioning in combination with an articulated alar rim graft placement created the desired contour of the tip, and opened the external valve.

On cadaveric costal cartilage

WONG

Russell Kridel's very detailed and long-term clinical series on cadaveric costal cartilage graft changed the landscape with respect to revision rhinoplasty in the United States.[34] His article was responsible for a "run" on costal cartilage stock through most of the United States. I myself do occasionally use cadaveric cartilage, but I reserve it for those patients who are older with less of a long-term time horizon, or in those patients whom I know have significant calcification. I do tend to get computed tomography scans on occasion of the thorax to evaluate potential calcification patterns. Although this study is excellent, it is only 1 study with few reports having this length of long-term follow-up. We really do not have a broad "crowdsourced" outcome with respect to how cadaveric costal cartilage will sustain itself over a very long time intervals. Thus, I am very reluctant to use it in young patients who may live 50 or 60 more years.

HAMILTON

I also occasionally use irradiated costal cartilage. Dr Kridel's study[34] has resulted in my slight increase in enthusiasm for using irradiated rib. Nevertheless, it is important to recognize that not all irradiated costal cartilage products are the same. There are several methods for processing and these variations may have an impact on the graft in the long term.[35–40] Institutional cost concerns frequently result in vendor or product changes. I am not confident that I can always count on getting the same product in the operating room. In contrast, autologous cartilage certainly comes from a predictable source and its longevity has been well-documented.[34] If I do decide to use irradiated rib in a patient, my criteria are similar to Dr Wong's. I avoid using it in younger patients and those who need structural support. In my experience, irradiated rib grafts placed under compression are more likely to resorb.

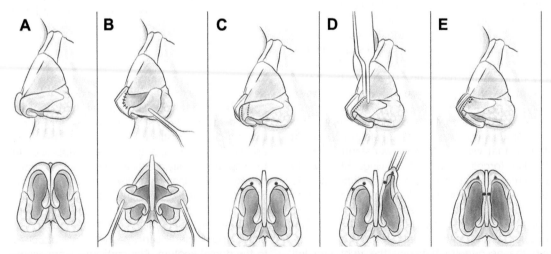

Fig. 16. Lateral crural tensioning. (*A*) Native tip cartilage architecture, (*B*) "boomerang" septal extension graft placement (may be side to side as well), (*C*) blue dots indicate position of native domes, (*D*) red triangles indicate new dome location created using a lateral crural steal, and (*E*) suture placement to septal extension. (*From* Foulad A, Vlogger V, Wong B. Lateral crural tensioning for refinement of the nasal tip and increasing alar stability: a case series. Facial Plast Surg 2017;33(3):317; with permission.)

FRIEDMAN

Irradiated rib definitely has a place in nasal surgery, but over time, mostly for practical purposes, I have come to rely on this material much less frequently. When I use irradiated rib, I remove the outer cortex and rely only on the inner cortex. I soak the carved segments of irradiated rib cartilage for 30 minutes or longer, and with this technique I find little warping or resorption. In the past, I relied on irradiated rib very frequently in hopes of reducing the morbidity associated with autologous rib graft harvest. As my experience with autologous rib harvest increased (owing to inconsistent availability of irradiated rib in the operating room), I have simply stopped asking for irradiated rib with any regularity. When a lot of strong structural support is needed (as when the majority of septal support needs to be replaced), I usually turn to autologous rib harvests. Additionally, I have come to appreciate ear cartilage as an outstanding graft material for both contour and structural support; laminating 2 pieces of ear cartilage with a small piece of septal cartilage or ethmoid bone provides excellent structural support when there is a need for additional grafting material.

On costal cartilage

WONG

Costal cartilage is the workhorse in most revision rhinoplasty operations when one needs to reestablish structure. I will harvest it readily. I know there has been some transition away from using only central balanced cross-sections, but I have no experience with this. That being said, I have used very thin lateral sections to reinforce the L-strut without issue. Incisions from costal cartilage have not been a real issue, and most of my patients will see a laser dermatologist in my group for resurfacing after surgery.[41]

HAMILTON

I have a fairly low threshold for using costal cartilage. It takes me less time to get cartilage from 1 rib than to get cartilage from 2 ears, and I can get more material. Patients also report less discomfort after rib harvest than compared with the ear. This might have more to do with the ear bolster and side sleeping. Nevertheless, if one avoids using monopolar cautery in the chest and does not cut the muscle, the discomfort after costal cartilage harvest is minimal. Also, with a careful subperichondrial dissection, the risk of a pneumothorax is very low.

FRIEDMAN

I use costal cartilage without hesitation when large amounts of strong structural supporting grafts are required, as when the entire septal cartilage is missing and there is not only a missing dorsal and caudal L strut, but there is no septum support whatsoever. Autologous rib would also be brought in for contracted skin that requires tremendous support to prevent wound contracture during the healing process (granulomatous polyangiitis), or in multiple-revised noses in which there is no septal or alar cartilage available to work with. In the vast majority of cases, however, including revision surgery, I do not find it necessary to harvest autologous rib. I generally rely on remnant fragments of septal cartilage and bone, and reinforcing these tissues with conchal cartilage grafts if necessary.

On auricular cartilage

WONG

I have become less reliant on auricular cartilage over the years, as my facility with rib has increased and my incisions have gotten a little bit smaller each year. I will use auricular cartilage, however, if the need is for volume and there is not a significant loadbearing role, and curvature is not too much of an issue. For me, this comes to play in terms of fashioning spreader grafts, and in primary rhinoplasty particularly in certain ethnic patients, quadrangular cartilage is inadequate. In these patients, I reserve quadrangular cartilage for septal extensions, and rim grafts.

HAMILTON

My order preference for cartilage donor sites is septal, costal, and auricular. I will use auricular cartilage for composite grafts and when a patient only needs batten grafts and I want to use the innate curvature of the concha. I will also use auricular cartilage for spreader grafts when the septum is inadequate, but this happens only rarely.

FRIEDMAN

Septal cartilage and bone is my first choice for grafting materials, followed by ear cartilage, autologous rib cartilage, and finally irradiated rib cartilage. If only a small amount of septal cartilage is available, I use it first for providing structural support for the nasal tip (the caudal portion of the "L-strut"). If that is all the septal cartilage available to me, I then rely on ear cartilage to support the dorsal aspect of the L-strut, generally using the ear cartilage as an extended spreader graft to help support the dorsum and the caudal septal replacement. Ear cartilage is my most common source for graft material in rhinoplasty.

On tissue engineering

WONG

This is the dream and grail for the rhinoplasty surgeon, and we are not there yet. Our colleagues in orthopedic surgery will use these products before we have the opportunity, and we will ride on their coattails.

HAMILTON

Tissue engineering is an encouraging development. However, I do question the practicality of growing a block of cartilage well In advance of surgery when the patient has already done that in their ribs.

FRIEDMAN

This is an exciting area of active research and I believe it will be available to us in our lifetimes. This will represent a tremendously positive step forward for our patients, and I cannot think of an operation that would be more suited to this development than rhinoplasty.

Question 7: What have you done differently over the past 5 years?

HAMILTON

In the last 5 years, there have been several changes in my grafting techniques. I am using more costal cartilage than auricular cartilage in patients who have an inadequate supply of septal cartilage. Beside the better quantity and quality of the cartilage, I have found that the rib harvest is significantly less painful than the ear. I am also making my grafts much thinner and more elastic. The periphery of the rib cartilage is supple and elastic, but still quite strong. Costal cartilage grafts do not need to be thick, brittle, and bulky.

FRIEDMAN

In the past 5 years, I have stopped using irradiated rib cartilage. This trend started as a practical matter, because it was difficult to get the graft material for some time, so I was forced away from irradiated rib cartilage. Autologous grafts quickly became a preference of mine over irradiated rib. I prefer autologous materials for a number of reasons. First, they are plentiful. Second, patients are more comfortable using their own body's materials rather than allografts or alloplasts. Finally, they work great. In the vast majority of primary rhinoplasty cases, I am able

to make do with the patient's own septal cartilage, and rearranging the lower lateral cartilages and the upper lateral cartilages.

WONG

In the past 5 years, I have stopped using for the most part columellar struts, shield grafts, and cap grafts. I have also moved away from lateral crural struts. My work horse approach when grafting is needed is to use the lateral crural tension technique and articulated alar rim grafts. I have trended toward using more costal cartilage rather than auricular, mainly because I can now section them very precisely into 1.0-, 1.5-, and 2.0-mm-thick specimens.

REFERENCES

1. Dziewulski P, Dujon D, Spyriounis P, et al. A retrospective analysis of the results of 218 consecutive rhinoplasties. Br J Plast Surg 1995;48(7): 451–4. Available at: http://www.ncbi.nlm.nih.gov/pubmed/7551522. Accessed September 12, 2017.
2. Bagheri SC, Khan HA, Jahangirnia A, et al. An analysis of 101 primary cosmetic rhinoplasties. J Oral Maxillofac Surg 2012;70(4):902–9.
3. Wee JH, Park M-H, Oh S, et al. Complications associated with autologous rib cartilage use in rhinoplasty. JAMA Facial Plast Surg 2015;17(1):49.
4. Moon BJ, Lee HJ, Jang YJ. Outcomes following rhinoplasty using autologous costal cartilage. Arch Facial Plast Surg 2012;14(3):853–76.
5. Cuzalina A, Qaqish C. Revision rhinoplasty. Oral Maxillofac Surg Clin North Am 2012;24(1):119–30.
6. Johnson CM, Toriumi DM. Open structure rhinoplasty. Philadelphia: Saunders; 1990.
7. Leary RP, Manuel CT, Shamouelian D, et al. Finite element model analysis of cephalic trim on nasal tip stability. JAMA Facial Plast Surg 2015;17(6):413–20.
8. Manuel CT, Leary R, Protsenko DE, et al. Nasal tip support: a finite element analysis of the role of the caudal septum during tip depression. Laryngoscope 2014;124(3):649–54.
9. Shamouelian D, Leary RP, Manuel CT, et al. Rethinking nasal tip support: a finite element analysis. Laryngoscope 2015;125(2):326–30.
10. Tjoa T, Manuel CT, Leary RP, et al. A finite element model to simulate formation of the inverted-V deformity. JAMA Facial Plast Surg 2015;1–8. https://doi.org/10.1001/jamafacial.2015.1954.
11. Gandy JR, Manuel CT, Leary RP, et al. Quantifying optimal columellar strut dimensions for nasal tip stabilization after rhinoplasty via finite element analysis. JAMA Facial Plast Surg 2016. https://doi.org/10.1001/jamafacial.2015.2261.
12. Daniel RK, Calvert JW. Diced cartilage grafts in rhinoplasty surgery. Plast Reconstr Surg 2004;

113(7):2156–71. Available at: http://www.ncbi.nlm.nih.gov/pubmed/15253210. Accessed September 12, 2017.

13. Tasman A-J, Diener P-A, Litschel R. The diced cartilage glue graft for nasal augmentation. Morphometric evidence of longevity. JAMA Facial Plast Surg 2013; 15(2):86–94. Available at: http://www.ncbi.nlm.nih.gov/pubmed/23634447. Accessed September 12, 2017.

14. Toriumi DM. New concepts in nasal tip contouring. Arch Facial Plast Surg 2006;8(3):156.

15. Hamilton G. Form and function of the nasal tip: reorienting and reshaping the lateral crus. Facial Plast Surg 2016;32(1):49–58.

16. Davis RE. Lateral crural tensioning for refinement of the wide and underprojected nasal tip. Facial Plast Surg Clin North Am 2015;23(1):23–53.

17. Ballin A, Kim H, Chance E, et al. The articulated alar rim graft: reengineering the conventional alar rim graft for improved contour and support. Facial Plast Surg 2016;32(4):384–97.

18. Goodrich J, Wong B. Optimizing the soft tissue triangle, alar margin furrow, and alar ridge aesthetics: analysis and use of the articulate alar rim graft. Facial Plast Surg 2016;32(6):646–55.

19. Apaydin F. Rebuilding the middle vault in rhinoplasty: a new classification of spreader flaps/grafts. Facial Plast Surg 2016;32(6):638–45.

20. Deroee AF, Younes AA, Friedman O. External nasal valve collapse repair: the limited alar-facial stab approach. Laryngoscope 2011;121(3):474–9.

21. Coordes A, Loose SM, Hofmann VM, et al. Saddle nose deformity and septal perforation in granulomatosis with polyangiitis. Clin Otolaryngol 2017. https://doi.org/10.1111/coa.12977.

22. Wang LL, Friedman O. Update on injectables in the nose. Curr Opin Otolaryngol Head Neck Surg 2017; 25(4):307–13.

23. Thomas WW, Bucky L, Friedman O. Injectables in the nose: facts and controversies. Facial Plast Surg Clin North Am 2016;24(3):379–89.

24. Johnson ON, Kontis TC. Nonsurgical rhinoplasty. Facial Plast Surg 2016;32(5):500–6.

25. Foulad A, Manuel C, Wong BJF. Practical device for precise cutting of costal cartilage grafts to uniform thickness. Arch Facial Plast Surg 2011;13(4):259.

26. Wilson GC, Dias L, Faris C. A comparison of costal cartilage warping using oblique split vs concentric carving methods. JAMA Facial Plast Surg 2017. https://doi.org/10.1001/jamafacial.2017.0163.

27. Fry HJ. The interlocked stresses of articular cartilage. Br J Plast Surg 1974;27(4):363–4. Available at:

http://www.ncbi.nlm.nih.gov/pubmed/4429815. Accessed September 17, 2017.

28. Tripathi PB, Elghobashi S, Wong BJF. The myth of the internal nasal valve. JAMA Facial Plast Surg 2017;19(4):253.

29. Kovacevic M, Riedel F, Wurm J, et al. Cartilage scales embedded in fibrin gel. Facial Plast Surg 2017;33(2):225–32.

30. Foulad A, Volgger V, Wong B. Lateral crural tensioning for refinement of the nasal tip and increasing alar stability: a case series. Facial Plast Surg 2017;33(3):316–23.

31. Seyhan A. Classification of spreader flap techniques. Facial Plast Surg 2017;33(4):453.

32. Kim JH, Wong B. Analysis of cartilage-polydioxanone foil composite grafts. Facial Plast Surg 2013;29(6):502–5.

33. Fuller JC, Levesque PA, Lindsay RW. Polydioxanone plates are safe and effective for L-strut support in functional septorhinoplasty. Laryngoscope 2017. https://doi.org/10.1002/lary.26592.

34. Kridel RWH, Ashoori F, Liu ES, et al. Long-term use and follow-up of irradiated homologous costal cartilage grafts in the nose. Arch Facial Plast Surg 2009; 11(6):378–94.

35. Menger DJ, Trenité GJN. Irradiated homologous rib grafts in nasal reconstruction. Arch Facial Plast Surg 2010;12(2):114–8.

36. Burke AJC, Wang TD, Cook TA. Irradiated homograft rib cartilage in facial reconstruction. Arch Facial Plast Surg 2004;6(5):334.

37. Martinho AC, Rosifini Alves-Claro AP, Pino ES, et al. Effects of ionizing radiation and preservation on biomechanical properties of human costal cartilage. Cell Tissue Bank 2013;14(1):117–24.

38. Vieira EH, Gabrielli MA, Okamoto T, et al. Allogeneic transplants of rib cartilage preserved in 98% glycerol or 70% alcohol into the malar process of rats: a comparative histological study. J Nihon Univ Sch Dent 1993;35(2):96–103. Available at: http://www.ncbi.nlm.nih.gov/pubmed/8410209. Accessed September 12, 2017.

39. Wee JH, Mun SJ, Na WS, et al. Autologous vs irradiated homologous costal cartilage as graft material in rhinoplasty. JAMA Facial Plast Surg 2017;19(3):183.

40. Wong BJF, Giammanco PF. The use of preserved autogenous septal cartilage in "touch-up" rhinoplasty. Arch Facial Plast Surg 2003;5(4):349–53. Available at: http://www.ncbi.nlm.nih.gov/pubmed/12873875. Accessed September 12, 2017.

41. Oliaei S, Nelson J, Fitzpatrick R, et al. Laser treatment of scars. Facial Plast Surg 2012;28(5):518–24.

Injectable Fillers
Panel Discussion, Controversies, and Techniques

Theda C. Kontis, MD[a,b],*, Lisa Bunin, MD[c],
Rebecca Fitzgerald, MD[d]

KEYWORDS

- Injectable fillers • Cannula • Tear trough • Injectable complications

KEY POINTS

- New fillers have been developed for circumoral lip lines and these are now incorporated into lip definition and volumization techniques.
- Injectors must be facile with both cannula and needle techniques for the accurate and safe placement of fillers.
- Facial rejuvenation techniques have advanced with the improved understanding of facial volume loss with aging and with the development of newer products designed for the midface.

Panel discussion

1. What is your approach to the perioral area and lips and has it changed with the introduction of new Food and Drug Administration (FDA)–approved fillers?

2. How do you evaluate and treat the lower lid/midface and how aggressive are you in filling those regions?

3. What is your opinion of cannulas versus needles?

4. What complications with fillers have you seen and how do you avoid them?

5. What role do fillers play in off-face treatment in your practice?

6. How have your techniques changed over the past 5 years?

With the introduction of Restylane in 2003, the filler revolution began. This hyaluronic acid (HA) filler was proved dramatically superior to the then gold standard, collagen. Over the past 15 years, new products have been developed to meet the needs of the injectors and combined with improved understanding of facial aging, previously neglected areas of the face can now be targeted with fillers.

In this article, specialists have been invited from oculoplastic surgery and dermatology to discuss their techniques and opinions for injections into the lower lids, midface, and lips. Cosmetic injectors will find the differing viewpoints from physicians in different academic fields will not only highlight differences in personal techniques and philosophies, but also reinforce that there are multiple approaches to analyzing and treating the aging face.

Disclosure: R. Fitzgerald acts as a speaker, trainer, and member of the advisory boards for Allergan, Galderma, and Merz. L. Bunin has nothing to disclose. T.C. Kontis is a member of the Speaker Bureau and injector trainer for Galderma and Allergan.

[a] Department of Otolaryngology-Head and Neck Surgery, Division of Facial Plastic and Reconstructive Surgery, Johns Hopkins Medical Institutions, Baltimore, MD, USA; [b] Facial Plastic Surgicenter, LLC, 1838 Greene Tree Road, Suite 370, Baltimore, MD 21208, USA; [c] Private Practice, 1611 Pond Road #403, Allentown, PA 18104, USA; [d] Private Practice, 321 N Larchmont Boulevard #906, Los Angeles, CA 90004, USA
* Corresponding author. Facial Plastic Surgicenter, LLC, 1838 Greene Tree Road, Suite 370, Baltimore, MD 21208.
E-mail address: tckontis@aol.com

Facial Plast Surg Clin N Am 26 (2018) 225–236
https://doi.org/10.1016/j.fsc.2017.12.008
1064-7406/18/© 2017 Elsevier Inc. All rights reserved.

Question 1: What is your approach to the perioral area and lips and has it changed with the introduction of new Food and Drug Administration–approved fillers?

BUNIN

Knowledge of the effects of aging on the perioral area anatomy has greatly changed the way I fill this area. It is not just about filling the lip but also about understanding the anatomy of the area and the effects of aging on each layer. I have a large percentage of older patients (60–80 years) and really see the effect of bone loss in this area. Patients come in complaining of the Popeye look after dental surgery, and I prefer to wait until they are done with their dental procedures before I inject these patients with filler, because the underlying anatomy can change. Understanding the superficial and deeper fat pockets around the mouth has also changed my approach considerably. Although my younger patients (<40 years) often desire very full lips, even overinflated lips, my older patients have always come in scared of having a duck lip look. Often by just filling the fat pockets around the lip, without even touching the lip itself, the lip appears fuller and less deflated because it is lifted into a more youthful position. My favorite fillers for the immediate perioral area and fine witches' lines around the mouth are the thinner fillers like Restylane Silk and Belotero. I use the thicker more cross-linked hyaluronic acid (HA) fillers and calcium hydroxyapatite for the oral commissures and the marionette lines and if I need more perioral lift in an older patient (although I may layer the thinner fillers over these for the fine lines and skin side of the vermillion border). In my older patients with more bone loss, I often end up reinforcing their jaw line with calcium hydroxyapatite for more support. And softening the muscular pull with a small amount of neurotoxin in the depressor anguli oris muscles (DAO), the mentalis, and some of the deeper perioral lines helps soften as well as prolong the effect of the fillers.

With my older patients, I often add filler or neurotoxin in stages, gradually building up the area. This accomplishes several things: it causes less swelling and faster return to normal and a gradual adjustment to their new baseline, with an appreciation of each level of improvement. These patients tend to be surgery-avoiding, more private ("I don't want anyone to know") and want to look rested and refreshed, not different. Yet, when they see the change in each stage, they are more inclined to try a little more on subsequent visits, including lifting the midface with filler.

The newest HA fillers, Restylane Defyne and Restylane Refyne, with XpresHAn Technology, have been wonderful additions for this area. There is much less swelling with these products, less bunching up of material and reportedly more natural-looking expressions with muscle movement. I find these new products are most useful in the perioral, marionette, and chin areas, where unconscious contraction of the perioral mimetic muscles can cause irregular lines and folds. These areas can be harder to treat without the use of neurotoxin, but some patients are either neurotoxin-phobic or are unhappy with loss of movement in this area. I have found the newer fillers more forgiving with added fill here.

When doing a consultation for lip enhancement, I evaluate each of the fat compartments, the lip lines, the vermillion border, the symmetry of the lip resting and smiling, and the shape of the lip and take baseline photographs in each position. Many patients do not realize they have asymmetries or that they look different when they smile or have an uneven amount of tooth showing in different positions. I discuss their concerns and desires, and I make recommendations based on all these. If they want a very full, inflated lip, I prefer Juvéderm and Restylane-L, filling the border and substance of the lip, taking care to reshape the lip as needed. I also like how I can use the newer softer fillers (Restylane Silk and Belotero) to smooth out the wrinkles in the lip itself without overinflating the lip.

I always give patients a hand mirror and ask them for feedback. I reserve a little filler at the end to use in case they think they want a little more in an area; otherwise, I place it where I think it is needed. They appreciate the artistry and the concern for symmetry. But if someone comes in wanting an overly inflated lip, I talk to them about facial balance and proportion and often show them how adding a bit of volume in the cheek may allow them to attain more beautiful balance with a larger lip.

My favorite fillers in each area are as follows:
- Perioral fine lines and volume loss just above and below lip: Restylane Silk, Restylane Refyne, and Belotero
- Vermillion border and for lip substance: Restylane-L, Juvederm Ultra, and Restylane Refyne
- Smoothing lip surface wrinkling: Restylane Silk
- Oral commissres: Restylane-L and Juvederm Ultra, or Ultra Plus
- Marionette lines and jugal grooves: Restylane Lyft, Restylane Defyne, Juvéderm Ultra Plus, and Radiesse

FITZGERALD

The evolution of my approach to the perioral area has been to be as mindful of the supportive structures in that area as of the lips themselves. Advances in understanding of the anatomy of aging in this area have provided more site-specific targets to achieve more natural-looking results. These targets include bony support in the anterior maxilla and pyriform aperture as well as the superficial and deep fat compartments of the lip and chin. Newer FDA–approved fillers give the ability to use more robust agents where a good deal of support is needed and softer smoother agents in the lips and oral commissures themselves.

The hallmarks of a youthful perioral region include a smooth transition from the cheek to chin, devoid of shadowing, and a phi ratio in the lower third of the face and the lips as well as the anterior projection and eversion seen in younger lips. In young faces with early aging, changes addressing the lips alone, as an isolated entity, often yield good results. In those further along in the aging process, however, this approach may yield suboptimal results by taking this area of the face out of harmony with its adjacent surrounding area. In the perioral area, the labiomental hollow (from loss of labiomental fat in compartments that have now been identified and visualized in CT images of cadaveric specimens treated with radiopaque dye) creates an upside-down U-shaped shadow that separates the lower lip from the chin and results in a labiomental fold, which creates a distinct shadow that typifies the frown. Treating just along the vermillion border of the lip exacerbates this separation (as well as effacing the sharp definition of this border). Targeted treatment in this fat compartment with fillers, such as Restylane Defyne or Vollure, re-establishes this support. Also, just as there is suborbicularis fat around the eye, there is suborbicularis fat of the perioral region, and the volume of this deep lip fat contributes significantly to the appearance of anterior projection and eversion seen in the youthful lip. I have found that Restylane Refyne, Juvéderm, and Vollure work well here. Loss of bony and soft tissue support contribute to deviation from the ideal phi proportions often seen with aging in the perioral area. Bony remodeling in the anterior maxilla and pyriform aperture may increase the nasolabial angle, decreasing the convexity of the midface and resulting in the appearance of a longer upper lip. Additionally, as labiomental fat as well as fat deep to the mentalis wanes, the mentalis muscle (which originates on the bone and inserts into the skin at the base of the chin) appears to pull up on the chin shortening this area.

Treatment in these areas that support the lips, rather than just the lips alone, results in a more natural-looking result.

Additionally, newer soft fillers, such as Restylane Silk and Volbella, allow the ability to add natural-appearing contour and shape to the lips.

KONTIS

When I assess patients for lip injections, I place them in 1 of 2 categories: lip volume enhancement or no volume enhancement with or without smoker's lines. These categories allow understanding the desires of a patient and help me select the ideal product.

For a patient who wants volume enhancement, I choose Restylane-L or Juvéderm Ultra or Juvéderm Ultra Plus. I find these products give good volume to the lips and, by injection of the vermillion, I can achieve nice definition and augment the lip roll. If these patients also have smoker's lines, I treat the vermillion and cross-hatch injections (with very small amounts of product to avoid a chimpanzee look or produce visible filler lines). In these patients, I also may consider Restylane Silk or Volbella to treat the fine lines. I like to elevate the oral commissures with filler, when necessary and I find I can achieve a nice lift with the Juvéderm Ultra, Juvéderm Ultra Plus, and Restylane-L products. I often add 2 units of onabotulinumtoxinA (Botox) to the DAO for severely downturned oral commissures.

Poorly injected Hollywood stars have given lip filler a bad name and I find many patients fear the overinjected lip look. For these patients who just want some smoothing out of their lips, Restylane Silk and Volbella are typically my next go-to products. I have issues with each, however—excessive swelling with Silk and only 0.55 mL of Volbella in the syringe.

Question 2: How do you evaluate and treat the lower lid/midface and how aggressive are you in filling those regions?

BUNIN

The midface is the key to facial rejuvenation. A young face has the triangle of youth: heart shaped, widest at the cheeks, and narrower at the chin. As bone, fat, and tissue are lost, the midface loses support and starts to sag and deflate, slowly transforming into an inverted triangle, which is heavier at the base. The lower lid elongates and may even pull away from the eye, there is a split in the malar fat pad, hollows appear in the cheeks, and jowls form.

Early in my career as an oculoplastic surgeon treating flaccid ectropions of the lower lids after strokes and Bell palsy, I discovered that lifting the cheek surgically restores the position of the eyelid. When I first started using Radiesse (it was Radiance then), I found that filling the midface immediately gave a more youthful look, despite other wrinkles and deep lines, because it restored the width and balance of the face. I presented the Voluma-R Lift (R for Radiesse) in 2006 and have filled the midface/cheek area with multiple fillers since then. The midface is really the starting point and focal point of true facial rejuvenation. Although a patient may come in concerned about jowls and marionettes, lifting the midface through reinflation with fillers reduced the jowls and marionette lines, allowing less filler to be needed in those areas.

Even nasolabial folds are less noticeable when the cheek is no longer falling and pushing onto the fold area. Patients may come in complaining of prominent nasolabial folds, but I explain to them how the shifting anatomy created the fold and remind them that even babies with chubby cheeks have nasolabial folds. So, filling the cheek may minimize or negate the need for filling the nasolabial fold.

The midface, cheek, paranasal area, and nasolabial fold are all a continuum, but special care has to be taken when approaching the eye area. The orbital area should not be viewed merely as an extension of filling the cheek. The skin here is the thinnest skin in the body, the vessels are superficial, and the tissues are delicate.

Volume loss, negative vector, extra skin, periocular pigment, postinflammatory hyperpigmentation, and lid laxity all need to be considered. Overfilling this area in the presence of excessive skin can make the wrinkling appear worse. Pigment spots hidden in the shadow of a tear trough can appear more prominent by inflating and stretching the area with filler. If the fat pockets are too protuberant, then filling around them can make the cheek appear too heavy, and patients are more likely to get a Tyndall effect in this area if some filler needs to be placed superficially to cover the edges. It is wise to test what may happen in this area by manual elevation of the cheek to see what happens to the lower lid and by stretching the skin in the tear trough area. If there is lid laxity, excessive skin and/or fat, or a lot of periocular pigment, then patients may be better served by having eyelid surgery and skin rejuvenation with skin care and/or lasers.

Filling the area around the eye should be thought of as divided into 2 areas: filling the true tear trough (defined as a depression centered over the medial inferior orbital rim between the palpebral and orbital parts of the orbicularis muscle) and filling the orbitomalar groove and periocular area. The true tear trough area has anatomic landmarks that may be affected as much by congenital anatomy as by aging. If photos of children's faces are examined, a visible tear trough is often found; if so, the, use of fillers will not completely efface the tear trough. The appearance of a tear trough deformity can also be exacerbated by having allergies. It is important to ask patients about allergies and eyelid swelling and to ask about eye rubbing. Patients with these conditions may have much more swelling after injections, more tendency for postinflammatory hyperpigmentation and bruising, and more fluctuation with sodium intake.

When filling the tear trough and periocular area, I use only thinner HA fillers, such as Restylane, Restylane Silk, and Belotero. I have also used Restylane Refyne in this area in a few patients known to have excessive swelling with HA's and have been happy with the results. I prefer not to use Juvéderm because it is more hydrophilic and more likely to cause a Tyndall effect. (The Tyndall effect occurs when HA is injected too superficially, leading to a bluish discoloration under the skin caused by the way the colloid particles scatter light.) I am less aggressive in these areas, preferring to use less filler and adding more if needed on a second visit. This area must be approached slowly, with care, and it is best to avoid overfilling and the resultant excessive swelling. HA fillers can last a long time in this area, and this is the most common place where I am consulted for hyaluronidase injections to correct overfilling and/or Tyndall effects. HA fillers should be injected deeply, onto the periosteum, in small aliquots, for the best results.

If a patient requires or desires cheek or midface enhancement, I do that prior to filling the periocular area, because elevating the cheek often reduces the amount of filler needed around the eye.

FITZGERALD

The manifestations of midfacial aging are largely due to changes in facial volume that transition the midface from a youthful convex platform dominated by highlights to an aged flattened platform segmented by shadows (concavities), as has been eloquently described by Glasgold.[1] The combination of volume loss and the effect of the underlying facial retaining ligaments contributes to the hallmarks of midface aging. Volume loss at the inferior orbital rim creates a concavity and overlying shadow, separating the lower eyelid from the cheek. In the anterior cheek, volume loss unveils a central hollow with its base tethered by the zygomatico-cutaneous ligament. Loss of deep cheek fat, which contributes to the anterior projection of the cheek, may worsen the nasolabial fold. Lateral cheek volume loss skeletonizes the zygomatic arch, creating a harsh submalar shadow. Hollowing of the temples interrupts the oval facial frame seen from continuous light reflection from the arc of the upper cheek and the temple. In the midface, augmentation of the medial aspect of the anterior cheek alone worsens the separation from the eye, upper lip, buccal area, and temple, often contributing to an unnatural appearance. Addressing the shadow group of the midface as a whole allows the creation of a unified cheek highlight with no separation between the cheek, the eye, and the upper perioral unit. Adding volume in the inferior orbital rim reunifies the lower eyelid and cheek segments. Softer fillers, such as Vollure, Volbella, and Restylane Refyne, work well in this area. A hydrophilic product like Juvéderm may cause an unwanted persistant edema. More robust products like Voluma or Restylane Lyft or Defyne may be visible through the thin overlying skin. Particulate collagen–stimulating agents like Sculptra (poly-L-lactic acid) or Radiesse (calcium hydroxylapatite) may clump in the orbicularis muscle, leading to nodules and should be avoided around the muscles of the eyes and lips. Volumization of the medial and lateral cheek should be addressed first, because support in this area may decrease (or even eliminate) the need for treatment in the tear troughs and nasojugal fold, especially in younger patients with good skin elasticity. Too much filler directly in the tear trough or nasojugal fold gives an odd topography to the face and is one of the most common novice errors. Additionally, because the lower eyelid skin has few appendages (and is, therefore, relatively see through), HA filler in this area is often visible reflecting light with a blue hue, commonly referred to as the Tyndall effect.

Filling the cheek, with a focus on both the medial and lateral deep cheek fat compartments, camouflages the zygomatico-cutaneous ligament depression and recreates a convex cheek with a strong highlight. Lesser volume is then needed in the area of the medial and lateral suborbicularis fat. Volume may need to be added to the zygomatic arch and lateral cheek when there is deficient lateral bony projection. Supraperiosteal injections done to create lift mimicking deep fat or bone can be done with more robust HA agents like Voluma, Restylane Lyft, and Restylane Defyne as well as Radiesse or Scupltra. Evidence from almost a decade ago supports the hypothesis of statistically significant bony remodeling in specific areas of the craniofacial skeleton with age, which may affect the draping of the outer soft tissues. A recent study measuring changes in 7 patients with a mean age of 61 years and CT scans on average 10.3 years apart showed that resorption was consistently present (100%) at the pyriform aperture and the anterior wall of the maxilla. Resorption was also noted at the superocentral (71%), inferolateral (57%), and superomedial (57%) aspects of the orbital rim.[2] Voluma and Sculptra are my products of choice when treating deeply around the pyriform aperture because they do not cause much swelling. I dilute 1 mL of Voluma with 0.5 mL of normal saline and administer it with a 26-gauge needle to allow for aspiration prior to injection in this area (although the reliability of aspiration is controversial). Recent studies of this pyriform space (also known as Ristow space) reveal it to be a large area with the angular artery running along the roof of the space, allowing for safe injections deeply along the bone.

Radiesse, Juvéderm Ultra Plus, Vollure, Restylane, Restylane Defyne, or Restylane Refyne can be used in the nasolabial fold area if it is not improved with the cheek injections alone.

Filling around the zygomatic arch is important to eliminate harsh shadows and restore youthful soft contours to the lateral cheek. The buccal region often needs to be addressed as it transitions the lateral facial contour of the zygoma into the lateral mandible. I have found that Sculptra or Vollure both work well in these areas.

KONTIS

In evaluating the midface, I separate the anatomy into lower lid, lateral cheek, and medial cheek, often using different fillers for each region. I am hoping that injectors stop referring to the lower lid volume loss as the tear trough deformity. When injectors were just starting to use fillers in the lower lids, very small amounts of filler were placed deep in the nasojugal groove. In my practice, I am now treating the entire lower lid area of volume loss over the entire extent of the inferior orbital rim, which may require excessive amounts of filler to achieve adequate volume restoration and smooth the junction from the lower lid to the midface.

When injecting the lower lid, I have a frank conversation with patients about the difficulty in achieving perfect results but how the lower lid hollows can certainly be improved. I also counsel patients who are not candidates for filler to the lower lids due to excessive fat herniation and would benefit more from a surgical fat removal. Patients who present for lower lid filler are told that they must be patient with the injections because I do not inject more than 1 mL of product along the inferior orbital rim at each visit. Appointments are separated by 2 weeks to 3 weeks and injections performed until I believe the results are the best I can achieve. Occasionally I have patients help improve their results by performing warm compresses to areas of irregularity. I usually select Restylane-L or Belotero for injection of the lower lids, because I find that the hydrophilic nature of Juvederm Ultra and Ultra Plus, as well as their occasional migration, can look like accentuated lower lid bags.

My treatment of the midface medially is a natural extension of treating the lower lid volume deficiency. With similar HA products, I extend injections to the anterior midface to improve this area if it appears flattened (as is the case with many Asian faces).

My approach to the lateral cheek radically changed after I attended a course given by Dr Mauricio deMaio. His technique is pulling the cheek back and depositing high lift (high G′) products, like Voluma or Restylane Lyft, to spot-weld the cheek laterally.[3] This technique revolumizes the malar cheek laterally and somewhat improves the nasolabial folds, jowls, and marionette lines. I have noticed that inexperienced injectors continue to fill just the nasolabial folds, marionette lines, and lips and ignore the midface or, worse, inject too medially in the midface. These injection techniques build out the central contours of the face producing a horse-like face or cherubic face, neither of which is aesthetically pleasing.

Question 3: What is your opinion of cannulas versus needles?

FITZGERALD

I like and use both for different areas of the face. I use 26-gauge needles with product diluted with saline (0.5 mL per 1 mL of filler) for supraperiosteal injections in the midface, usually Voluma or Restylane Lyft, and 26-gauge needles with Juvederm Ultra Plus diluted with saline (2 mL saline per 1 mL of filler) deep to the temporalis muscle in the temple. I occasionally use 27-gauge or 30-gauge needles in the lips or oral commissures but more often use cannulas, and I use cannulas everywhere else with HA filler or Radiesse. I use a 25-gauge 1.5-in needle with Sculptra.

The biggest concern with injections, of course, is safety. Other important concerns are precision and the degree of swelling and bruising. In my experience, precision is possible with both needles and cannulas. One recent study using fluoroscopically controlled injection of material found that when using needles the injected material is more prone to migrate to more superficial layers, whereas using cannulas resulted in the material remaining in the targeted layer of intended application, leading them to the conclusion that using cannulas results in higher precision of placement than using needles.[4]

Bruising may be a little less with cannulas, although experience, knowledge of anatomy, and speed of injection also play an important role. Certainly experienced injectors can treat whole faces with a needle without causing bruising. I sometimes choose needles over cannulas in areas of previous scarring, such as the lateral cheek in a post-facelift patient, if it is difficult to glide the cannula. I do use cannulas exclusively in patients who cannot stop their anticoagulants.

Regarding safety, ischemia, necrosis, and even, albeit rarely, blindness, cerebrovascular accidents, and nonthrombotic pulmonary embolism have occurred with cosmetic injection stemming from vascular occlusion. Blunt cannulas may reduce, but not eliminate, risk, because they can still penetrate vessels with sufficient force. Some practitioners aspirate prior to injection to reduce risk with both cannulas and needles. Aspirating blood is indicative of intravascular needle placement and warrants removal of the needle and repositioning. Failure to aspirate blood, however, is not a guarantee that the needle is not in a vessel, because the bevel of the needle may be suctioned against the vessel wall, preventing aspiration. Recommendation of aspiration as a risk reduction strategy is controversial because many injectors believe that aspiration may not be reliable (or even possible) with thin needles and thick gels. Product diluted with saline or lidocaine (0.5 mL per 1-mL filler) and/or used with larger gauge needles may make this possible but has not been studied. I have refluxed blood on aspiration on many occasions over the years using Sculptra with a 25-gauge needle.

Unanimously accepted risk reduction practices include any and all measures that could prevent an inadvertent intravascular injection of filler material, especially large amounts under high or sustained pressure. Because the volume and speed of filler material inadvertently injected in a vessel may play a role in the severity and prognosis of an occlusive event, it is prudent to use small amounts per pass through a constantly moving needle or cannula tip to minimize the risk of injecting significant volumes into a vessel. Smaller syringe size may facilitate this. It is important to avoid placing a bolus of material unless the needle is in a known avascular area (eg, on bone). Additionally, avoiding high-pressure injections is of paramount importance. Unintended high-pressure injections may occur inadvertently from pushing against a small blockage in a needle or cannula. Therefore, if any resistance is felt on injection, removal of the syringe to clear (or replace) the needle or cannula prior to reinjecting the patient is prudent. In areas of rich vascular anastomoses, such as the central face, even a very small amount of volume under high pressure can be devastating if it reaches the retina. It is important to know the location and depth of facial vessels as well as the common variations of vascular patterns. Scheuer and colleagues[5] presented an excellent review of facial danger zones.

Finally, a sharp needle can injure an artery from every direction. Perpendicular alignment of the needle is advised to approach an artery. With a needle, it is believed that parallel insertion increases the chance of residing within the arterial segment compared with perpendicular insertion. Creases form over underlying arterial vasculature (such as the nasolabial crease over the angular artery), and can be used as a topographic landmark to guide needle placement. In contrast, when using a cannula, a recent cadaveric study by Tansatit and colleagues[6] found that insertion of a cannula parallel to the artery could not create arterial injury, leading these investigators to conclude that parallel insertion is, therefore, safer when using a blunt cannula. This may be negated if the artery has a tortuous path, the cannula hits a bifurcation in the artery, or if the artery is fixed to the tissue by a fibrous septum from previous scarring (trauma, surgery, or injections). Again, be aware that during a blinded insertion of a cannula to reach the target area, the injector cannot discriminate the sensation at the cannula tip between the resistance of a fibrous septum and the resistance of an artery that is held in place by a fibrous band. This presents a high chance of arterial injury. When resistance is encountered, reinsertion to pass around the resistance is a better choice than a forceful insertion to pass through the resistance. Never force the cannula through a resistance—change direction or reinsert.

Prompt recognition of an embolic event, of course, enables prompt management, and prompt management can hasten resolution and minimize undesired sequelae. Immediate blanching or a dusky color consistent with ischemia should be treated as such as soon as possible with hyaluronidase to the entire dusky area (because the embolus may be distal to the original site of injection).

BUNIN

To someone with a hammer, everything looks like a nail. Both cannulas and needles are useful when placing filler, and success with either depends on technique, the filler used, the area to be filled, and the length and gauge of the needle or cannula used. In general, needles are easier for beginner injectors to understand exactly what level they are in and for anyone when precise placement is needed in small areas or for fine lines. If used carefully, slowly, and under magnification, risks of bruising are minimized. Slow injection and pulling back on the syringe before injecting minimize risks of injecting into a vessel. Proponents of cannulae use suggest that there is less risk of both of these, but poor technique mitigates any advantages. Use of cannulas has a longer learning curve, and it can be more difficult to gauge the level of placement. It is also harder to pass through prior filled areas where some scarring has occurred and to be as precise in small areas, such as fine tuning the nasal tear trough and treating superficial fine lines.

Currently, I like to use cannulas for filling the lower face and jaw line and for the lateral and temporal fat pockets. I often use smaller cannulas for filling the periorbital area but may touch up the true tear trough area (nasal) with a 30-gauge needle for more precision. Longer cannulas can be harder to manipulate but work well for filling the lower face and up into cheek hollows. Thicker products require larger gauge cannulas, which can also add to tissue trauma if not handled with expertise.

When I do use needles, especially for the lips, I like to use longer needles than are often included with the syringe in the box of filler. I regularly use a 30-gauge 1-in needle or a 28-gauge $^{3}/_{4}$-in needle for the lips, depending on the thickness of the filler used. Fewer needle pokes means less swelling, less eosinophilic response, less bruising, easier gauging of filler results, and potentially faster recovery. For the marionettes and jawline, I usually use a 1.25-in needle near the jawline, allowing for a wide access from 1 focal point.

KONTIS

I believe that injecting with a cannula is like using a fire hose to deposit filler. It may be fine for large depositions of product, but I like to inject product at varying depths and do not believe I have the fine control of a needle when I am using a cannula.

The proponents of cannula use believe they improve the safety of injections and diminish bruising, but there is no literature supporting that cannula use is really safer and that belief can provide a false sense of security when injecting.[7] I would argue that a large deposition of product can externally collapse a vessel even if it does not embolize it. I have also had patients bruise after cannula use because I have to use a needle to initiate the tract into the skin. In addition, it does require some pushing and shoving to get the cannula to tract in the skin, whereas the needle usually glides freely. I have on occasion caused bruising with a cannula due to the shoving I needed to perform to move it subcutaneously. I think those who say that cannulas do not cause bruising are mistaken. A 1-entry point with a needle and fanning out the product can also be used in similar way that a needle is used. Needles are more precise in my hands. I also believe that I end up wasting more product with a cannula because I deposit more out of the syringe, I believe I use less product in each area with a needle. That said, this is not an all-or-nothing answer. In certain cases, I do prefer a cannula, such as for injection of the upper lid A-frame deformity and along the jawline. The skilled injector should be facile with either technique.

In my opinion, if an injector injects slowly and carefully and knows the anatomy, then the injector is a safe injector, regardless of using a needle or cannula. I think possibly the safety in cannula use is that it results in slower injections, a process that increases safety. I believe that with needles, I can achieve safe and minimally traumatic injections with slow, meticulous injections, even in patients who are anticoagulated.

What is interesting to me about those who advocate 100% cannula use for safety is that they all agree that there are areas where cannulas cannot be used well, like the lips, lower lids, fine lines, and so forth.

Question 4: What complications with fillers have you seen and how do you avoid them?

FITZGERALD

My practice has been almost 100% injectables for many years now (other doctors in the office use lasers and devices) so I have seen my fair share of complications of my own as well as many referred in by other physicians.[8] Fortunately, a vast majority of adverse events are not severe, although they are fairly commonplace. They are mostly secondary to the injection itself or to the injector and include transient swelling, erythema, and bruising as well as various technical errors leading to suboptimal outcomes. These include errors in the amount of volume used, depth of placement, location of placement, and/or product choice for a specific location. Obviously, with any preventable complication, avoidance is preferable to management and becomes possible with a thorough knowledge of anatomy, adequate practical training, and shared experience. Bruising is one

of the most common patient complaints because they believe they are signing up for a no downtime procedure and do not want to field questions about it from family, friends, and coworkers. Bruising may be minimized with the use of blunt tip cannulas as well as with slow injections with smaller aliquots of the product. Some practitioners believe that bruising may be reduced by using arnica, aloe vera, or vitamin K creams. Use of an AccuVein AV300 (AccuVein, Cold Spring Harbor, New York) near-infrared device to image veins otherwise not readily visible from the skin surface has helped me reduce the incidence of bruising in my practice. Additionally, pulsed dye laser at 24 hours to 48 hours may hasten the resolution of bruising.

Severe filler complications are fortunately rare. These include occlusive vascular events, as discussed previously, as well as late and delayed inflammatory events, which may represent infectious (biofilm) or immune-mediated events.

In cases of vascular occlusion, as discussed previosuly, prompt recognition enables prompt management, and prompt management can hasten resolution and minimize undesired sequelae.

Immediate blanching or a dusky color consistent with ischemia should be treated as such as soon as possible with a high dose of hyaluronidase (300–600 units) to the entire dusky area (because the embolus may be distal to the original site of injection) at intervals of 30 minutes to 60 minutes until cleared. Adjuvant therapy includes aspirin and antivirals and antibiotics. Hyperbaric oxygen can also be used (particularly if the occlusion is a non-HA product and cannot be dissolved).

In cases of delayed inflammatory reactions, a definitive, conclusive explanation of the mechanism of action of these events—including whether they are infectious or immune mediated or both—remains elusive, making prevention and treatment challenging. Cultures (for bacteria and atypical mycobacterium) can be obtained but are often negative. Biopsy may confirm the presence of a granulomatous reaction. If the product is HA, hyaluronidase can be used to dissolve the product. If a lot of inflammation is present, the lesions must be incised and drained but often recur intermittently over time with each flare a little less than the previous one; 5-fluorouracil is an antimicrobial and antimetabolite and has been used successfully to resolve these reactions. It may be prudent to avoid treatment in patients with active autoimmune disease or poor dental hygiene. Additionally, thorough facial cleansing and preparation (avoiding the use of tap water, which can be contaminated with atypical mycobacterium) are strongly recommended.

BUNIN

Careful technique and thorough knowledge of facial anatomy are imperative for good outcomes and for avoiding most complications. Understanding the characteristics and ideal placement of each filler are also critical, as is managing patient expectations. It is important to separate mild side effects of any injection, such as bruising and swelling, which are transient (although aesthetically displeasing) from true complications, which can be sight threatening and disfiguring.

Swelling can be due to the hydrophilicity of the filler, from Juvéderm, which is the most water-loving (it routinely swells), to the newer Restylane Defyne and Restylane Refyne, which hardly swell at all. Using ice before and after injection and using longer needles with fewer sticks (less immunoglobulin E–mediated reaction) and/or using a cannula can all help to minimize swelling. Bruising can be minimized by having the patient stop all blood thinners, including aspirins, nonsteroidal anti-inflammatory drugs, vitamins, fish oil, flaxseed oil, gingko balboa, and green tea 10 days to 2 weeks before treatment, and by using loupes or a vein locator to avoid vessels. Pulling back on the needle prior to injecting and slow injection are helpful, and, if bleeding occurs when the needle or cannula is withdrawn, simply applying pressure and ice for several minutes can go a long way toward minimizing a bruise. I also like to use sublingual arnica pills preinjection for sensitive patients and when injecting Sculptra, and I use K-Derm Cream on the area postinjection. I use this on all of my eyelid surgery patients and find it resolves the bruise in half the time.

Other common complications that are mild include lumpiness and small noninflamed nodules, poor placement, inadequate volumization, poor aesthetic result, and asymmetry. Most of these can be avoided or minimized with careful preprocedure assessment, careful injection technique, and proper depth of placement of each filler. I always photograph the patient pretreatment, point out any natural asymmetries of the area before filling, and give the patient a hand mirror to assess the results before I finish the injections so they can point out any asymmetries or areas of concern, which I can address right then.

Moderate and more troubling complications include Tyndall effect, painful nodules (biofilm), and true granulomas. Tyndall effect is most common around the eyes and is more common with Juvéderm, so I never use that product in this area. I have many patients sent to me because of this, and careful use of hyaluronidase can dissolve the HA filler. Although some injectors advocate using large doses of hyaluronidase and totally removing the filler and starting again with a different filler with deep placement, I find most patients are happier if I reduce the overfill and leave some filler in place. I use very small aliquots and see the patient back in 2 weeks, at which time I may use more hyaluronidase to further reduce the filler or may touch up the area with properly placed filler if a patient wishes.

Nodules that are palpable but not visible are usually due to clumping of material in muscle fibers or having had some calcification of a bruise. Reassuring patients that these nodules are not dangerous and will gradually resolve with massage or on their own is usually treatment enough. I have had a few patients develop nodules with Sculptra, which were treated with intralesional injection of Kenalog. I have only had to excise 2 nodules, which occurred in the suprabrow area in a very thin patient, and they healed beautifully. These all occurred early in my career, and I now dilute the Sculptra with 9 mL to 10 mL of sterile water and inject deeply, especially in the temples, and avoid the suprabrow area.

Fortunately, I have not had patients develop any red, painful nodules, but if I did I would immediately consider infection or a biofilm as the cause and would use oral and topical antibiotics. It is imperative that thorough cleansing of any area be done prior to breaking the skin surface with a needle.

Finally, there is the remote possibility of more severe complications of injecting into a vessel with tissue necrosis and even blindness. Slow careful injections with aspiration on the needle should minimize this risk but does not completely eliminate it. If any blanching is seen, or a patient complains of pain out of proportion to the injection, stop injecting immediately and assess for complications. In addition to using warm compresses and massage if vascular compromise is suspected, every injector should be prepared with a crash cart of aspirin, nitropaste and hyaluronidase.

KONTIS

Fortunately, I have had few serious injectable complications and none with permanent sequelae; however, these patients tend to be remembered in vivid detail.

My first complication occurred while I was performing a nasal dorsum augmentation on a patient who had undergone 2 previous rhinoplasties and I was trying to improve some mild supratip depression. My injection with HA was too superficial and his nose immediately blanched (as did I); then the skin became mottled and purple. With the immediate use of massage, warm compresses, hyaluronidase, and nitropaste, he went on to completely recover. I am now extremely careful injecting operated noses. I reflux before every nasal injection and make sure I am injecting into the avascular preperiosteal or preperichondrial plane.

The 2 other serious complications I have seen (1 was my patient and 1 was referred to me) were due to vascular injury to the superior labial artery. The key to injecting these patients is rapid diagnosis and treatment. I think the photos of patients with necrosis of facial tissues needing hyperbaric oxygen treatments are those who went home after their injection with an undiagnosed vascular injury.

Every injector should have a protocol to follow for suspected vascular injury.[9] My protocol is to stop injections if a blanching is noted and to massage and apply warm compresses. Generally, this improves the majority of cases. For patients who do not respond to these measures, I proceed with oral aspirin (for the patient), hyaluronidase injection to the site of suspected vascular occlusion, and topical nitropaste (kept in the office.)

I have seen a few nodules with products, which generally resolve with massage or injection with hyaluronidase or Kenalog. I did have 1 patient develop severe nodules over her entire face 2 years after Sculptra injection. These were firm, lumpy nodules that gave the face almost a cottage cheese appearance. She was taking an antimetabolite (mercaptopurine) for inflammatory bowel disease, which may have been associated with this complication. The nodules all appeared at the same time and responded to intramodular injection of 5-fluorouracil with Kenalog.

Question 5: What role do fillers play in off-face treatment in your practice?

BUNIN

Aging tends to show in the face, neck and décolletage, and most patients seek rejuvenation in these areas, but aging hands give away a patient's true age. Hand volumizing and rejuvenation have been a big part of my practice for more than 10 years. I love using Radiesse to volumize the hands, and find results can last 2 years or more. I use intense pulsed light (IPL), fractionated lasers, and medical-grade skin care to reduce pigmentation and change the skin texture. Recently I have used Restylane Defyne to volumize hands because there is minimal swelling with this product but have no data on longevity yet.

Sculptra has been used at high dilutions for off-face rejuvenation for the hands and décolletage but my experience is limited, and I have no experience with fillers for buttocks augmentation.

KONTIS

As patients become more savvy about injectables, they are starting to ask about off-face injections. I find that treatment of the dorsum of the hands in women and men is becoming more popular.

In hand dorsum injections, I prefer Radiesse because the 1.5-mL syringe is usually enough to treat both hands. The filler is placed in depot fashion between the muscle tendons and massaged to fill in the furrows. It is important to explain to patients that the veins in their hand may look less prominent but still be visible.

I have experimented using Volbella as a skin booster in the anterior neck to improve crepey skin; however, there seems to be some persistent lumpiness for several weeks postinjection.

I do not find patients request fillers much to treat the neck and décolletage. I have had some success with treating the necklace lines and décolletage with neurotoxins but have not used fillers in these areas.

FITZGERALD

I use a fair amount of Sculptra in the décolletage. I am not treating buttocks or knees, but many practitioners have obtained nice results with this product in those areas.

I also use a fair amount of Radiesse in the dorsal hands.

Question 6: How have your techniques changed over the past 5 years?

BUNIN

My techniques now involve more volumizing, layering, combining treatments, using cannulas as well as replacing areas of facial volume loss to restore a more youthful appearance. Doctors have stopped looking at wrinkles and sagging skin in isolation and are considering how volume loss in 1 area affects others, how muscle pulling plays a role, and how bone loss affects the supporting framework. Filling the temples makes a large impact on the brows and upper eyelids; assessing the masseter, jawline, preauricular area, and chin and combining well-placed filler with neuromodulators can give subtle but definite changes in proportion that appear more beautiful. I am using more neuromodulators in the lower face and neck than ever before. Treating the platysmal bands, performing a Nefertiti neck lift, treating overactive masseter muscles, and relaxing muscles to enhance the effect of filler have become routine. I am using a lot more Sculptra to support the underlying foundation of the face in a global fashion, then layering fillers over that in specific areas. Rejuvenating the skin with medical-grade skin care, facials, peels, microdermabrasion, IPL, and/or lasers is important, but I now have far more laser and light options available.

The biggest challenge is deciding how much to do and in what order. This depends on patients' desires, budget, timeline, and anatomy and whether they are also having eyelid or brow surgery. If a patient flies in from out of town, or has a big event in a month, I do as much as I can in 1 sitting. Otherwise, I prefer to rejuvenate the patient in stages.

In general, I like to start almost everyone on medical-grade skin care because healthy skin responds better to any treatment, even when doing neurotoxin or a little bit of filler.

I routinely perform neurotoxin and filler on the same day if they are done to different areas and sometimes in the same areas. I am more cautious using neurotoxin to elevate the lateral brow if I have used a large volume of filler around the brows and temples because I have seen fluid influx into this area carry the neurotoxin inferiorly and cause a mild ptosis.

If IPL, skin-tightening lasers, or other noninvasive procedures to the face are being done, I perform those first and then do filler and/or neurotoxin. I not do invasive procedures and fillers or neurotoxin on the same area on the same day but may do them in a distant area (eg, fill lips and also laser resurface around the eyes). I routinely combine laser resurfacing with eyelid surgery and suggest neurotoxin to the crow's feet and lateral eyebrow, either 2 weeks or more before the surgery or a few weeks after the lasered areas have healed. This enhances the surgical results and allows better skin remodeling by reducing muscle traction on the area.

I try to convey to my patients how investing in themselves earlier gives long-term results. Taking care of their skin, putting collagen "in the bank" through tissue stimulation with Sculptra and skin-tightening modalities like the Titan laser, softening muscle contraction lines with neuromodulators, and reinflating early with fillers can stave off the need for surgery and can actually slow the aging process: 60 is the new 40, and 80 is the new 60. Even though I am a surgeon, surgery is not the only answer. I tell them I am like a seamstress—I can sew a beautiful garment, but I cannot make leather into silk, and how the garment drapes depends on the underlying tissue. So, skin care,

fillers, neuromodulators, and good health all play a role in maintaining a rested youthful appearance, and the time to start is now.

FITZGERALD

Over the last five years, I have become better at recognizing how to approach some problems and in recognizing which patients I can or cannot help. This recognition and targeted correction of currently recognized specific anatomic deficiencies are constantly improving because of the wealth of studies available. These gains in knowledge sometimes enable site-specific correction of areas primarily responsible for the development of downstream markers of aging to give predictable targets for predictable and natural appearing results. There is still so much to learn and understand; however, advances and innovations in technology have given faster and more efficient ways to both gather and share information and are accelerating understanding of this complex process. This has led to a paradigm shift in the way the changes seen in the aging face are both perceived and approached. The answer to the question of whether the face sinks or sags has become a "yes" to both, as aging is beginning to be seen as a complex and interdependent interplay between all structural layers culminating in the collapse of 3-D construct. Newer understanding of volume loss as a critical component of facial aging and the integration of volume replacement into the surgical and nonsurgical therapeutic algorithm will greatly enhance the ability to address the loss with site-specific corrections to achieve optimal and natural-looking results in a predictable manner.

At the same time, the products used to achieve these corrections are constantly improving. I feel lucky to practice in a time of renaissance in this field of cosmetic injectables.

KONTIS

I am certainly using more syringes of fillers in a treatment than I used 5 years ago. In the past, injectors were taught to focus on the nasolabial folds, marionette lines and lips. Now not only is there a better understanding of facial volume loss but also the injectable products themselves are being created to give more options for "total correction."

When I assess a patient for injectables, I now evaluate the entire face. Do the temples look hollow? If so, I may consider Sculptra, Restylane Lyft, or Voluma to those regions. If the hollowness extends into the preauricular regions, I may prefer Sculptra because lumpiness of the HA fillers is difficult to avoid in that area. I address midface volume next and find I am injecting the actual nasolabial folds either not at all or with much less product once the cheeks have been volumized. Then I work inferiorly to the circumoral region, where I now like to use Restylane Refyne. I find this filler takes almost no skill to use and produces fantastic, smooth results.

I am also more aggressive with lower lid injections. I treat the entire lower lid crescent to maximal correction using not more than 1 syringe of filler at a time. Where in the past 1 area tended to be focused on, I think now injectors are looking at reshaping the face and trying to restore the heart-shaped, volumized youthful look.

I often inject 1 side of the face and stop to show patients the difference between the treated and untreated sides. I point out to them where I injected the filler to create the volumization and lift. I would say that 99% of patients are "wowed" by the results they see in the mirror.

As new products are developed with increasing longevity, I believe patients are more willing to purchase multiple syringes at a setting, especially once they see how total facial rejuvenation improves their appearance. Combined with neurotoxins, many call this a "liquid facelift," although it is neither liquid nor a facelift. I may start telling my patients this is "panfacial rejuvenation with injectables."

ACKNOWLEDGMENTS

T.C. Kontis thanks L. Bunin and R. Fitzgerald for their thoughtful and thorough responses to these questions and hopes readers improve their injectable knowledge from this discourse.

REFERENCES

1. Glasgold MJ, Glasgold RA, Lam SM. Volume restoration and facial aesthetics. Facial Plast Surg Clin North Am 2008;16(4):435–42.

2. Karunanayake M, To F, Efanov JI, et al. Analysis of craniofacial remodeling in the aging midface using reconstructed three-dimensional models in paired individuals. Plast Reconstr Surg 2017;140(3):448e–54e.

3. de Maio M, Rzany B. Injectable fillers in aesthetic medicine. 2nd edition. Berlin: Springer-Verlag; 2014. p. 89–92.

4. Pavicic T, Frank K, Erlbacher K, et al. Precision in dermal filling: a comparison between needle and cannula when using soft tissue fillers. J Drugs Dermatol 2017;16(9):866–72.

5. Scheuer J, Sieber D, Pezeshk R, et al. Anatomy of the facial danger zones: maximizing safety during soft-tissue filler injections. Plast Reconstr Surg 2017;139:50e.

6. Tansatit T, Apinuntrum P, Phetudom T. A dark side of the cannula injections: how arterial wall perforations and emboli occur. Aesthetic Plast Surg 2017;41(1):221–7.

7. Yeh LC, Fabi SG, Welsh K. Arterial penetration with blunt-tipped cannulas using injectables: a false sense of safety? Dermatol Surg 2017;43(3):464–7.

8. Fitzgerald R, Bertucci V, Sykes J, et al. Adverse reactions to injectable fillers. Facial Plast Surg 2016;32: 532–55.

9. Dayan SH, Arkins JP, Mathison CC. Management of impending necrosis associated with soft tissue filler injections. J Drugs Dermatol 2011;10(9):1007–12.

Orbital Fractures

Kris S. Moe, MD[a,b], Andrew H. Murr, MD[c], Sara Tullis Wester, MD[d,*]

KEYWORDS

- Orbital fractures • Orbital reconstruction • Endoscopy • Exophthalmometry

KEY POINTS

- Anatomic, rather than volumetric, reconstruction leads to improved outcomes in orbital reconstruction.
- Endoscopic visualization improves lighting and magnification of the surgical site and allows the entire operative team to understand and participate in the procedure.
- Mirror-image overlay display with navigation-guided surgery allows in situ fine adjustment of the implant contours to match the contralateral uninjured orbit.
- Precise exophthalmometry is important before, during, and after surgery to provide optimal surgical results.

Panel discussion

1. What is your preoperative management protocol for patients with orbital fractures?
2. What factors you consider in deciding on surgery for these patients?
3. What are your preferred surgical approaches for orbital fractures?
4. What is your preferred technique for fracture repair?
5. How do you manage these patients postoperatively, and what surgical outcomes do you expect?
6. How have your techniques changed over the past 5 years?

Question 1: What is your preoperative management protocol for patients with orbital fractures?

MOE

My policy for evaluating patients with orbital injury is to first proceed with the Advanced Trauma Life Support protocol for evaluation and resuscitation. After evaluation to confirm hemodynamic stability and rule out intracranial injury, a complete craniofacial examination is performed and a maxillofacial CT scan is obtained with 0.625-mm–cut thickness. Three-dimensional reconstructions are performed when there are fractures involving bones adjacent to the orbit, such as the zygoma or maxilla. Visual acuity is checked, and range of motion of the extraocular musculature is analyzed, looking for signs of entrapment. Visual fields are checked. Color vision is evaluated (in particular, red). Direct and consensual pupillary functions are checked (swinging flashlight test) to rule out an afferent pupillary defect, which suggests injury to the globe or neural pathways. An ocular examination is performed with attention to conjunctival edema, hemorrhage, and hyphema. Globe position is noted, and exophthalmos, if present, suggests the need for tonometry to check intraocular pressure (IOP) and careful evaluation of the CT scan for a retrobulbar hematoma. An ophthalmology consult is requested to rule out injury to the globe.

Disclosure: The authors have nothing to disclose.
[a] Division of Facial Plastic and Reconstructive Surgery, Department of Otolaryngology, University of Washington School of Medicine, Seattle, WA, USA; [b] Department of Neurological Surgery, University of Washington School of Medicine, Seattle, WA, USA; [c] Department of Otolaryngology–Head and Surgery, University of California, San Francisco, School of Medicine, San Francisco, CA, USA; [d] Oculofacial Plastic and Reconstructive Surgery, Orbital Surgery and Oncology, Bascom Palmer Eye Institute, University of Miami Miller School of Medicine, 900 NW 17th Street, Miami, FL 33136, USA
* Corresponding author.
E-mail address: SWester2@med.miami.edu

Facial Plast Surg Clin N Am 26 (2018) 237–251
https://doi.org/10.1016/j.fsc.2017.12.007
1064-7406/18/© 2017 Elsevier Inc. All rights reserved.

The primary condition that may require urgent treatment by surgeons who are not ophthalmologists is retrobulbar hematoma. Retrobulbar hematoma is a collection of blood in the retrobulbar space, which may evolve rapidly. The accumulation of blood may lead to increased IOP and anterior displacement of the globe, thereby placing the optic nerve under tension. This is a critical condition analogous to a compartment syndrome with arterial and venous occlusion and obstruction of ocular perfusion. Initially reversible, if left untreated, it can result in blindness. If there is concern for elevated IOP in a patient with suspected retrobulbar hematoma, emergent canthotomy and cantholysis are indicated, particularly in the setting of decreased visual acuity. The signs and symptoms are described previously. If this is suspected, emergent ophthalmology consultation should be obtained, canthotomy and cantholysis are performed, and consideration is given to administration of intravenous steroid and mannitol or acetazolamide and return to the operating room to obtain hemostasis and resect the hematoma.

A somewhat less urgent condition is the pediatric white eye fracture. This refers to a trapdoor fracture that entraps an extraocular muscle. The relative elasticity of pediatric bone allows the fracture to open and then collapse on orbital contents, possibly diminishing the blood supply to the structures involved. The patient often has nausea and vomiting and may also have bradycardia. The term, *white eye*, refers to the lack of visible external signs of trauma that is common in these patients; my policy is to repair these fractures within 12 hours to avoid permanent damage to the entrapped muscle. Injuries to the globe and optic nerve are given priority over the treatment of orbital fractures, and fracture repair is not undertaken until definitive clearance is provided by an ophthalmologist.

Patients with orbital fractures without evidence of globe or optic nerve injury are given follow-up clinic appointments 7 days to 10 days after injury. I do not prescribe antibiotics, although for patients with extensive periorbital edema, I consider a short course of oral steroids. Ice packs are recommended for 48 hours to 72 hours for symptomatic relief. By waiting 7 days to 10 days after injury to evaluate the patient in clinic, the majority of traumatic edema will have subsided, allowing more accurate assessment of globe position and condition; initial complaints of diplopia may have resolved, and occasionally patients who presented without diplopia will develop diplopia due to change in globe position. For patients with other significant craniofacial fractures, in particular those that involve occlusion or major fractures of the zygoma and maxilla, the decision to operate may be made earlier to incorporate the care of those fractures.

MURR

My current work-up of orbital fractures has had a nuanced evolution over the past 2 decades. Patients can be divided into approximately 2 categories: those patients with an isolated orbital fracture or an orbital fracture with a zygomatic complex fracture and those patients with more extensive injuries and higher-impact trauma that have associated midface fractures like Le Fort fractures or nasoethmoid complex fractures. Often patients with higher-impact trauma are brought in to the care setting through the trauma center and have a higher likelihood of associated injuries. These patients are often managed in close partnership with the neurosurgery service. Patients with isolated orbital fractures, however, are often more ambulatory and may come to the office setting for care or through less acute entry portals, such as an urgent care practice. The basic work-up involves a detailed history and physical examination. Time of injury should be determined and mechanism of injury. Physical examination keys on pupillary reaction to light, extraocular motility, and sensory nerve evaluation, especially the fifth nerve. Entrapment, if suspected, heightens the acuity of the need for repair. White eye fractures, especially in the pediatric population, should be suspected if a patient has severe pain or nausea when extraocular motility maneuvers are attempted. This is important because it is one of the true emergencies associated with the evaluation of orbital fracture patients. In the white eye fracture, orbital contents are entrapped in a minimally displaced trapdoor or green stick fracture that is easy to miss on imaging. Yet, the occulocardiac reflex can produce bradycardia, nausea, and syncope in a patient with an orbit that appears otherwise uninjured. Typically, the inferior rectus is tethered, and surgery to release it as soon as possible is required. The presence of hyphema or pupillary eccentricity should be specifically ruled out during the physical examination. I have learned to use a Naugle exophthalmometer to compare the 2 eyes with regard to projection and enophthalmos. The Naugle instrument also helps me to assess the globe position and, therefore, guides my assessment of postoperative results. The key study for any orbital fracture or suspected orbital fracture is a fine-cut axial, coronal, and sagittal CT scan. These days, most patients have already had this study done; 0.625-mm cuts are preferred to completely assess the orbital floor in my practice, but the image guidance protocols released by manufacturers generally allow 1.0-mm to 1.5-mm scans.[1] I do not find 3-D reconstructions critical to the work-up, however. Another reason the fine-cut scan is preferred is because the fine-cut algorithm is necessary for image guidance equipment. With regard to preoperative treatment, I typically do not recommend antibiotics or corticosteroid medication. Finally, there is the question of the need for formal ophthalmologic evaluation. In my book the answer is...always. I always ask my ophthalmology colleagues to do a baseline examination of a patient. They are able to assess the retina and provide invaluable preoperative documentation. The consultation is not often emergent; however, it is necessary. Furthermore, in the event of intraoperative questions or difficulty, the ophthalmology service will not be surprised regarding patients and their treatment path.

WESTER

When patients present with concern for orbital fracture, several tests are performed. Visual acuity, IOP, and pupillary size and response are always checked prior to dilating the pupil. Alterations in pupillary size may be suggestive of inferior oblique damage (as the parasympathetic fibers to the ciliary ganglion, which ultimately innervate the sphincter pupillae, travel along with the inferior oblique muscle). Alterations in pupillary response are concerning for traumatic optic neuropathy or other causes of damage to the optic nerve. This must be documented preoperatively, so that a preexisting traumatic optic neuropathy is not mistaken for an intraoperative complication. A full ophthalmologic examination is performed to rule out hyphema or iritis, lens injury, globe injury, retinal trauma (Berlin edema, commotio retinae, retinal tears or detachment, and in cases of a rapid moving foreign body sclopetaria), foreign body, optic nerve compression or traumatic optic neuropathy, retrobulbar hemorrhage, or evidence of significant intraorbital emphysema. These issues should be addressed prior to fracture repair, except for cases of inferior rectus entrapment with an oculocardiac reflex. The oculocardiac reflex (bradycardia, nausea, and syncope) portends a risk of fatal arrhythmia and patients who exhibit these signs should be closely monitored and urgently repaired. Checking and careful documentation of extraocular motility are of paramount importance. Patients are also checked for hypesthesia of the infraorbital nerve and enophthalmos (I use the Hertel exophthalmometer [see **Fig. 2**]). Many times in the acute setting enophthalmos is not seen due to edema, but as the edema subsides, enophthalmos can occur, which can be both functionally and aesthetically significant for a patient. Subtle clues to enophthalmos are a deeper superior sulcus on the involved side or a relative ptosis.

In general, imaging is performed as soon as possible and emergently in children with concern for oculocardiac reflex. I recommend thin-sliced high-resolution orbital helical CT with contrast with 1-mm to 2-mm cuts through the orbit with both axial and coronal views. This allows for short acquisition time, reduced motion artifact, less radiation exposure, and better detection of soft tissue entrapment. The size of the fracture, location of the fracture, and relationship of extraocular muscles and critical orbital contents to the fracture are assessed. The adjacent sinuses and bony integrity of the skull base are also assessed and any foreign body should be identified. The identification of the presence or absence of a posterior ledge is a critical landmark to assess on preoperative imaging. The absence of a posterior ledge to the orbital floor requires different implant techniques. The integrity of the inferomedial bony strut should also be assessed, because loss of the strut portends a worse prognosis in terms of globe displacement and dysmsotility. As discussed later, the amount and location of soft tissue herniation are also important in determining which cases are more likely to need surgical intervention. Assessment of the size and caliber of involved extraocular muscles is also important, and the presence or absence of extraocular muscle or retrobulbar hematoma should be well documented. In addition, rounding of the inferior rectus on CT scan can be an indicator of greater soft tissue disruptions,[2] which may be associated with greater risk of enophthalmos and fibrosis leading to worse motility outcomes. In patients who have had previous surgery, vertical elongation of the muscle may suggest tethering of the muscle to a previous placed implant and may be an indication for reoperation in cases with clinical symptoms.

In the acute setting (ie, when a patient presents after acute fracture), I recommend avoiding nose blowing and strenuous activity, particularly if there is any evidence clinically or on imaging of intraorbital emphysema. For fractures of the medial wall and floor of the orbit, antibiotic therapy is initiated. In addition, for acute trapdoor fractures, antiemetics may be required and close monitoring of heart rate should be performed. I generally do not use steroids preoperatively.

Question 2: What factors you consider in deciding on surgery for these patients?

MOE

The decision whether or not to operate is typically made when a patient returns to clinic 7 days to 10 days after initial injury, as noted previously. Our decision to operate is made by answering a straightforward question: Is there an alteration of form or function? If not, there is rarely an indication for surgery. The primary decision to operate is thus typically based on the presence of diplopia that is not improving and is not expected to resolve, with the goal of concomitant aesthetic improvement.

A major criterion that was popular in the older literature was the presence of a fracture that involved more than 50% of the orbital floor. I do not consider this for several reasons; it is not possible to see the entire floor on a single CT image, so calculating the percentage of floor fractured is challenging; the percentage of floor fractured does not correlate with position of the globe; and the percentage of floor fractured fails to predict the presence or severity of diplopia (**Fig. 1**). I do not use CT scans for determination of entrapment, because this is a clinical diagnosis and true muscle entrapment (rather than fat) is rare.

Determination of alteration in form or function is made is several ways. The patient typically notes any disturbance of these. A change in globe position is often described by the patient as a change in eyelid position. Enophthalmos leads to decreased vertical aperture (distance between the upper and lower lids), whereas exophthalmos increases the vertical aperture. Determination of the contribution of globe position versus lid position to the perceived change in appearance can be challenging at times, particularly in cases of significant trauma to the eye lids. For this reason, and for comparison to the normal orbit and outcomes analytics, I perform Hertel exophthalmometry (**Fig. 2**) on all patients on presentation, at the beginning and conclusion of surgery, and at each follow-up.

Normal globe position is usually within 2 mm of the contralateral side. Although it is uncommon for a patient to elect to have surgery for enophthalmos without diplopia, for patients who do have diplopia, the prospect of also improving globe position reinforces their decision to proceed. For patients who appear to have globe position or orbital volume changes not expected from the location or

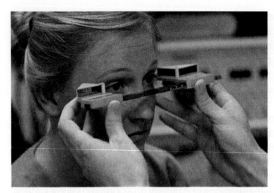

Fig. 2. Hertel exophthalmometry. The exophthalmometer is placed on the lateral orbital rims, and the projection of each globe to the corneal apex is measured through a prism.

severity of the fracture, it can be helpful to ask patients to see a premorbid photograph, such as a driver's license. Patients are often unaware of preexisting orbital asymmetry, and attempts to create symmetry will be unsuccessful and possibly deleterious.

Precise measurement of diplopia requires the use of prisms, which can be time consuming. We, therefore, estimate the position of onset of diplopia relative to central gaze using 15° intervals up to 45° in each direction (eg, 30° vertical, 15° right lateral). I record and repeat this analysis at each clinic visit.

Patient age is important. Young children without entrapment are commonly observed, unless the fracture is severe. I have noted spontaneous improvement of bone position in some children followed over time. There is no cutoff beyond which a patient is too elderly to undergo repair; the elderly may be more at risk for falls or other accidents with a small amount of diplopia. Other considerations, such as employment, are important. College and professional athletes require special consideration both in the decision to operate and whether surgery can be delayed to the off-season.

The timing of surgery is highly important. Rather than attempting to repair the fracture within a week of injury, as was common in the past, unless muscle entrapment is demonstrated on forced ductions, we delay surgery for a minimum of 1 week after injury. This allows much of the edema to resolve, bringing the globe more nearly into a settled position. This may allow minor diplopia to resolve or, less commonly, may lead to the delayed onset of diplopia. It is important for these changes to occur before deciding on repair. Furthermore, the repair can be performed more precisely, with less retraction pressure on orbital contents, when the majority of the edema has resolved. Although excessive delay of repair may allow displaced orbital contents

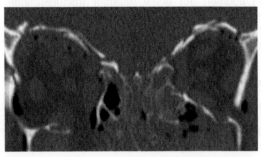

Fig. 1. Severe bilateral 4-wall orbital fractures with no diplopia; patient declined repairs.

to adhere to the sites into which they herniate, the use of delicate dissection under endoscopic visualization provides good results for fractures that occurred even years earlier.

MURR

Indications for surgery to repair orbital fractures are fluid. In some cases, the presence of associated fractures strongly tips the balance toward surgery. For isolated orbital fractures, however, I think there is some disparity regarding need for treatment and observation to sort out which patient actually needs surgical treatment. Yet, in an inner-city trauma practice, with poor patient reliability and discordant follow-up potential, a treating physician may have a limited window to recommend and carry out surgery. The question becomes, Are there any specific indicators that heavily push the decision toward intervention rather than watchful waiting? Certain points remain central to operative decision making. These points are (1) entrapment, (2) size of the floor defect, (3) increased intraorbital volume, (4) enophthalmos, and (5) diplopia. Entrapment is perhaps the least controversial of the indications. Although I perform forced duction testing in the operating room, I rely on my ophthalmology colleagues to perform forced duction testing, if indicated, in the ambulatory setting. The size of the defect is also a prominent indicator. As a rule of thumb, greater than 50% loss of the orbital floor on CT scan supports a decision to proceed surgically. In addition, if the inferior rectus is rounded and oriented vertically, the fracture portends future enophthalmos that require eventual correction.[3] The term, *increased intraorbital volume*, is a bit loose. As a general concept, if the volume of the fractured orbit is 10% greater than the unfractured side, this is a reason to proceed with surgical correction. Measurement of enophthalmos is usually objective either using an exophthalmometer.

Although persistent diplopia is a reasonable indication for orbital floor repair, immediate diplopia alone as an indication for surgery is not always a reliable reason to support surgical intervention because diplopia from an orbit fracture may resolve on its own without the need for specific intervention over time. I have a high threshold for exploring and repairing medial orbital wall fractures because in my experience few medial orbital wall fractures cause long-range problems. Orbital roof fractures are also able to be managed expectantly in a large percentage of cases. This is especially true in children where orbital roof fractures are more common than in the adult population. A review by Redett in 2014 noted that of 159 orbital

roof fractures in their database, the vast majority could be managed conservatively. Vertical dystopia occurred in less than 1% of patients and was associated with large fractures (>2 cm³) or fractures with inferior displacement or blow-in fractures. The investigators noted that they would have a lower threshold to repair if the patient required a craniotomy or other frontal bone repair due to the injury sustained.[4]

Timing of repair of orbital fractures is controversial in all cases except cases of entrapment. This includes the white eye fracture, where there are minimal signs of trauma, including on CT imaging, but there is entrapment of the orbital contents such that there is limitation of upward gaze and possibly occulocardiac reflex findings, such as nausea. These entrapment cases should be surgically approached as soon as possible. Most cases of orbital fracture repair, however, are elective. The ideal timing in my mind is at the 10-day to 2-week point in general. This allows for edema to resolve, for imaging to be obtained, and for ophthalmologic consultation to be accomplished and being sure that repair is necessary. Some clinical investigators have found that the need to accomplish repair can be made distantly from the acute injury.[5] If based on enophthalmos and diplopia, many floor fractures that are repaired in my current algorithm might not actually need to be repaired. One article by Harris divided orbital floor fracture into 2 groups, A and B. A-group fractures were minimally displaced but B-group fractures had herniation of orbital contents into the maxillary sinus and rounding of the inferior rectus muscle. Harris recommended that B-group fractures should be repaired within approximately 3 days because they found a worse motility outcome in the fracture group, which underwent delayed repair. The A-group group (except for the white eye fracture) could be safely repaired at approximately 2 weeks postinjury.[6] Nevertheless, Dal Canto and Linberg[7] looked at approximately 50 patients and found no difference between an early repair group fixed by 2 weeks and a delayed repair group fixed between 2 weeks and 4 weeks. There are reports in the literature that show good repair results for patients with diplopia or enophthalmos quite distant from the injury.

WESTER

Several factors are considered when deciding on whether surgery is indicated in cases of orbital fractures. My practice has shifted over time, because I have found that many patients heal to their satisfaction without surgical intervention. Surgery in the acute setting is indicated for fractures that show clinical signs of entrapment. I do not use imaging to guide my assessment of entrapment, because entrapment is a clinical diagnosis. Imaging is always performed, however, as discussed previously, to guide fracture repair approach and assess for damage to other ocular or adjacent structures. My general indications for surgical interventions include diplopia, fracture larger than 50% of the floor, and enophthalmos, but, as discussed later, in borderline cases I find that orbital soft tissue herniation is a good indicator of risk of late enophthalmos.

For pediatric patients with clinical evidence of entrapment, rapid repair of the fracture is indicated, preferably within 24 hours to 48 hours. In the event of the oculocardiac reflex, the urgency is even greater. Generally speaking, a 2-week observation period before surgery is advised for fractures greater than 50% of the floor, enophthalmos greater than or equal to 2 mm, or diplopia, to allow posttraumatic edema to subside and to ensure the diplopia does not resolve on its own.

Clinical findings are the number 1 indication for surgical intervention. I have seen cases of radiographic findings not consistent with clinical findings, and I always base my intervention on the clinical picture. This is especially true for trapdoor fractures. Although some surgeons advocate for MRI as superior to CT in showing soft tissue herniation in these cases,[8] I advocate that clinical diagnosis is the most accurate and assists in more rapid repair of the fracture (which is associated with improved outcomes). In addition, although studies have shown a much better concordance between radiographic findings and clinical symptoms in the adult population (likely due to the more common finding of larger fractures with herniation of tissue), I have had several cases of patients undergoing sinus and dental procedures with small fractures that were not easily identified radiographically.

I believe that many fractures spontaneously heal with conservative management, and studies have demonstrated neobone formation and reduction in orbital volume with time. Therefore, for smaller fractures without significant soft tissue herniation and without clinical symptoms, I do not recommend surgical intervention. In borderline cases, I find observation appropriate, because many stabilize/improve and those that do not achieve good surgical results even if surgery is delayed for several months.

I also believe it is important that for patients with significant comorbidities and no meaningful vision from the involved eye, orbital fracture repair may not be indicated. As with all clinical decision making, a clear analysis of the risks and benefits in each surgical case is essential—which is another reason I advocate for preoperative ophthalmologic evaluation. A patient's career and hobbies can also play a role. For example, many patients are not bothered by diplopia in extreme upgaze, but a young professional cyclist may find this disabling and thus opt for earlier surgical intervention.

All patients should have this testing performed prior to surgery because many orbital traumas have concomitant ocular trauma that may need to be treated. If a patient has an occult ruptured globe, this sometimes is missed on imaging and pressure placed on the globe intraoperatively can lead to disastrous expulsion of intraocular contents. Although these cases are rare, the possible morbidity to patients is significant. In addition, a preoperative examination ensures that a preexisting condition is not mistaken for a surgical complication.

The fracture dimensions and location are critical to assess and often determine outcome. Posterior medial floor fractures with significant soft tissue (and inferior rectus) herniation may behave in many ways similarly to trapdoor fractures and intervention should be performed earlier to achieve optimum results. I find that imaging signs of changes in muscle contour and location of tissue herniation are helpful guides as well. Significant loss of anterior and medial floor, particularly if the strut is involved, is more likely to lead to late enophthalmos when there is soft tissue herniation.

Question 3: What are your preferred surgical approaches for orbital fractures?

MOE

After a patient is under general anesthetic, I perform exophthalmometry to check the position of the globe relative to the normal side. The procedure is begun by placing ophthalmic lubricant over the cornea of both eyes, and placing a temporary tarsorrhaphy suture in the contralateral eyelids over the lateral limbus, allowing both pupils to be visualized for comparison as needed. I prefer not to use corneal protectors because they must be removed to check pupil size, reactivity, and shape. The pupil must be checked carefully at the beginning of the case and regularly throughout the procedure to determine if any changes occur, which might indicate excessive retraction of the orbital contents.

My choices of incision and approach are based on the location and extent of the fracture. For an isolated fracture of the floor of small to moderate size, I use a transconjunctival inferior fornix approach. This is chosen over a preseptal approach because it leaves a protecting layer of fat on the lower lid and prevents lid malposition, in my experience. For a larger posterior floor fracture involving the orbital apex, or one that extends to involve the medial wall, I continue the incision into a precaruncular approach and typically perform a lateral canthotomy and canthopexy to prevent excessive lid retraction and optimize exposure.

For a medial wall fracture, I use a precaruncular approach[9] and extend it into an inferior fornix approach as needed. I also use this approach for ethmoid artery ligation and optic nerve decompression. For a lateral wall fracture, I use a lateral retrocanthal approach[10] with or without lateral canthotomy and cantholysis. Isolated fractures in this region are rare; the lateral wall is usually repaired in conjunction with zygomaticomaxillary complex or skull base/cranial fractures.

Orbital roof fractures are approached through an upper blepharoplasty incision, unless the fracture is a component of a frontal bone fracture that requires a coronal approach. These fractures often include an element of brain injury, and the indication for surgery is primarily to remove segments of bone that are protruding down into the levator and superior rectus muscles and occasionally to evacuate subdural or retrobulbar hematoma. If the fracture is not comminuted, I reposition the bone; if there are multiple fragments, I remove them and place a layer of resorbable polydioxanone (PDS) sheet, 0.25-mm thick, between the dura and orbital contents to prevent scarring of orbital contents to the dura and maintain compartmentalization.

When access to the orbit has been achieved, the periorbita is then incised and lifted off the orbital bone. A subperiosteal dissection plane is created, and a malleable elevator is placed for gentle elevation of the orbital contents, creating an optical cavity for endoscopic dissection. Once a cavity of sufficient size has been created, a segment of thin silastic sheet can be placed between the retractor and orbital contents for protection.

Endoscopic dissection has major advantages for orbital surgery[11] (**Fig. 3**). These include image magnification and superior illumination, with visualization on monitors that allow the entire surgical team follow the case. In addition, less retraction of orbital contents is required for the narrow, cylindrical optical cavity than is needed for the wider funnel-shaped approach of an open procedure. The primary dissection instrument is a suction Freer elevator. Before retrieving the orbital contents out of the fracture site, dissection proceeds around the fracture until the periosteum is elevated as much as possible off the adjacent bone. This allows visualization of the adjacent anatomy and maximal access to the herniated orbital contents. For more extensive fractures, as the orbital apex is approached, surgical navigation is used to confirm instrument location and distance from the optic nerve and posterior aspect of the fracture. After this dissection is completed and full visualization and comprehension of the anatomy is obtained, restoration of displaced orbital contents back into the orbit is performed. For medial wall and floor fractures, this involves freeing the orbital structures from the ethmoid and maxillary sinuses, respectively. Care must be taken to do this as gently as possible, restoring all of the orbital fat without damaging the muscles or neurovascular structures.

MURR

I began my career with an approach that was basically a cosmetic blepharoplasty approach to the orbit. This was a subtarsal or midlid approach via a skin-muscle flap. This approach was lower on the lid than a subcilliary approach, which had more potential for lid malposition, especially ectropion. The idea of lowering the incision from the subcilliary position was so that the subciliary pretarsal orbicularis oculi muscle remained untouched. This was believed to improve the complication rate. The incision was begun in a lateral crease and the dissection was taken down through the lateral orbicularis oculi and to the periosteum of the bone of the frontal-zygomatic buttress. Stevens scissors were then used to bluntly dissect the orbicularis oculi from the orbital septum using a hand-in-glove technique. Dissection is only carried as medially as the inferior lacrimal punctum. Once this tunnel is created, the scissors are turned so that the inferior tine is inside the tunnel that was created and by closing the scissors, the skin and muscle are incised all at once, turning the skin-muscle flap down. This is a beautiful technique that is extremely quick and gives excellent access to the entire orbital rim. The periosteum can then be incised and the floor dissected with a Freer. I think that most of my colleagues today prefer 1 of 2 transconjunctival techniques: either the preseptal approach (with or without a canthotomy) or the trans-septal direct technique through the fornix of the conjunctival fold. In a patient with eyelid creases, however, the midlid approach does an excellent job. I also use transconjunctival incisions. These are especially useful in youthful patients with no lid creases. The one I have used most is the preseptal approach with a canthotomy. I start the incision with the canthotomy and then use the same hand-in-glove dissection technique used in the midlid surgery to split the skin and muscle from the orbital septum and the conjunctiva from the inside of the lid. Access to the orbital rim and orbital

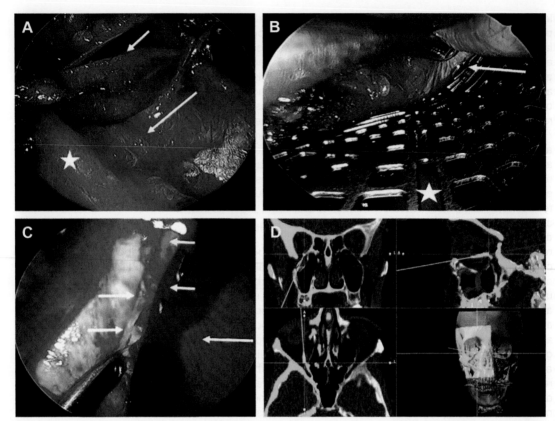

Fig. 3. Endoscopic repair of floor and medial wall fractures, right orbit. (*A*) Endoscopic view of fracture right orbital floor and medial wall; (*star*) infraorbital nerve; (*long arrow*) depressed floor fracture; and (*short arrow*) ledge of normal bone at orbital apex. (*B*) Endoscopic view of titanium mesh orbital implant; (*star*) infraorbital nerve seen through implant; and (*arrow*) elevator raising periorbita over posterior aspect of implant. (*C*) Endoscopic view of superior aspect of the medial wall with PDS sheet (*long yellow arrow*) lining the titanium mesh (*short yellow arrow*) resting on the bone of the lamina papyracea, where it joins the skull base (*green arrow*) inferior to the anterior and middle ethmoid arteries (*upper white arrow* and *lower white arrow*, respectively). (*D*) Navigation guidance to check position of orbital implant against the surgical plan of the normal contralateral orbit (*green*) superimposed over the fractured orbit (*white*); navigation probe resting on the implant represented by blue line.

contents is excellent. For closure, I use one 2-0 clear nylon to reposition the canthal tendon and close the skin of the canthotomy with 6-0 fast absorbing gut. No sutures are used in the conjunctiva itself. Lid malposition complications in this approach are more of the entropion type, which can be irritating to the cornea if they occur. As discussed previously, I do not usually find a need to surgically correct medial orbital wall fractures. The 2 main approaches, however, are the transcaruncular approach and the classic Lynch incision. The access of the Lynch incision is unparalleled and quick. To prevent webbing, I incorporate a running W-plasty into the classic Lynch incision. I have found that in all but young patients that it heals imperceptibly. This approach gives direct access to the lacrimal sac, which is preserved. Following the frontoethmoid suture line with a Freer or Cottle elevator, the anterior ethmoid artery can be controlled with

clips and transected. That frontoethmoid suture is also an excellent landmark for the level of the skull base. For a large medial wall fracture that is worthy of approaching and repairing surgically, I think that the exposure afforded by a Lynch incision for placing a large implant into the medial orbit is outstanding. Roof fractures would be approached using a superior lid blepharoplasty approach or perhaps a coronal approach if the frontal bone, frontal sinus, or anterior cranial fossa needed to be accessed. Currently, I use image guidance on orbital fractures. The scans are the same scans used for the sinus image guidance protocols. The set-up for image guidance does not take much time, but the image guidance probe at the end of the case can assure that the placement of the implant material is adjacent to whatever posterior ledge remains. I do not have easy access to intraoperative imaging, so real-time image guidance is the next best thing. I also have easy ability to pull the endoscopic sinus surgery set at any time that it is needed and can do it at a moment's notice. It is usually in the room but not opened because I do not always use the equipment. It must be emphasized that it is critical to accomplish a forced duction test at the beginning of the case, prior to wound closure, and after wound closure. Any catch or resistance must be investigated and corrected at the time of the surgery.

WESTER

My preferred surgical approaches for floor and medial wall fractures include the transconjunctival approach to the floor and transcaruncular or swinging eyelid approach for the medial orbit. A lateral canthotomy is generally not needed for floor and medial wall fracture repair. Prior to the incision, I check forced ductions. A Frost suture is placed through the lower eyelid and helpful for inferior traction intraoperatively and then affixed to the forehead postoperatively to reduce the risk of postoperative eyelid retraction. I also use intra-operative corneal protectors. My conjunctival incision is made just below the tarsus with monopolar cautery and blunt dissection with cotton tipped applicators anterior to the orbital septum down to the orbital rim is performed easily. Once the periosteum is opened and lifted off the floor, the fracture and important surrounding landmarks, such as the infraorbital nerve inferiorly, should be identified. In addition, if inferior or medial rectus or inferior oblique muscle is swollen or hemorrhag-ic, this should be assessed and documented. In these cases, even with proper implant placement, the forced duction testing may still reveal asym-metric resistance and portends a worse prognosis. The transcaruncular incision is a vertical incision through the caruncle with manual palpation of the posterior lacrimal crest and dissection of the periosteum off residual lamina posteriorly. This al-lows rapid access to the medial wall of the orbit. The same principles of fracture repair are used for each fracture location.

In terms of surgical approach, I do a fair amount of surgical planning in more complex cases to pro-vide landmarks of normal anatomy to guide my dissection. I use a hand-over-hand approach with manual reposition of herniated tissue starting from places of normal anatomy. Direct visualiza-tion is paramount to ensure that no mucosal tissue is pulled up into the orbit and that all herniated orbital tissue is appropriately repositioned. I some-times use a silicone sheet as a barrier in addition to the malleable to maintain previously dissected tis-sue within the orbital cavity and prevent this from obstructing my surgical view. I have not found intraoperative imaging or navigation systems necessary, although for complicated cases they may be beneficial. In these cases, I typically use premade customized implants based on preoper-ative imaging and these provide navigation land-marks. In addition, implant position is checked to ensure no incarceration of ocular tissue below the implant. I also always check preimplant and postimplant placement forced ductions. I have had to reoperate several cases where the referring doctor did not document forced ductions (and these patients had persistent entrapment or teth-ering). I also soak my implants in gentamicin prior to placement. In cases of fixation required, I fixate with self-tapping screws. In some cases, glue may be placed under the anterior edge of the implant to fixate it, although this is usually not necessary.

For closure, I use 4-0 vicryl and perform meticu-lous closure of periosteum. I close conjunctiva with several buried, interrupted 6-0 plain gut su-tures. For the rare cases of a traumatic incision in the lower lid, I use this as access to the floor and close with either 6-0 fast-absorbing plain gut or 7-0 nylon.

Question 4: What is your preferred technique for fracture repair?

MOE

Before beginning the reconstruction, the orbital contents must be delicately and completely freed from the fracture site. The periorbita should be lifted circumferentially around the fracture over an area large enough to provide stable seating of the implant. For extensive fractures involving the lateral floor, it may be necessary to transect the contents of the inferior fissure to allow proper implant place-ment. Contrary to the superior orbital fissure, which contains critical neurovascular structures that must be spared, the inferior fissure transmits fibrovas-cular tissue and minor sensory nerves that can be sacrificed without notable sequelae. This should be performed with meticulous bipolar cautery to prevent delayed hemorrhage.

Once the fracture site has been fully prepared, an implant of choice can be placed. For fractures of the medial wall and floor I used to shape the implant from flat titanium mesh; preshaped im-plants are now readily available that conform approximately the shape of a typical orbit, which are much easier to use and require less fitting. The implant is placed into approximate location, then positioned meticulously under endoscopic visualization.

Before the operation begins, a nurse or resident uploads the navigation CT scan into the system and creates a mirror-image overlay (MIO) template[12] (see **Fig. 3**D). This superimposes the image of the normal orbit over the fractured orbit as a guide for proper positioning of the implant. While accessing the fracture site, standard navigation views are used. After placement of the implant, the navigation is switched to the MIO view. A navigated suction or pointer is then passed over the surface of the implant to compare the actual implant position with the surgical plan. The position of the implant is then optimized, and contoured in situ using a small right-angled probe (Browne hook). After final positioning and contouring, the implant can be fixated, if desired, with a self-drilling screw typically placed in the thicker bone of the orbital rim. Unless the fracture is so large that it is difficult to stabilize the implant, I usually do not use screw fixation. As a last step, I line the entire surface of the implant with resorbable 0.25-mm thick PDS sheeting. This serves as a glide surface against which the orbital contents can easily slide as well as preventing herniation of orbital contents through the small gaps in the mesh. After the implant resorbs, it typically leaves a thin fibrous tissue layer that continues to function in similar fashion.

For fractures of the lateral wall and roof of the orbit, the primary goal is to remove bone that is impinging on orbital contents. These fractures rarely cause volumetric changes of the orbit, and the load-bearing type of titanium implant used for the floor and medial wall is not typically necessary. Even with extensive loss of orbital roof bone, if pulsatile exophthalmos occurs it usually resolves in 1 week to 2 weeks.

The question often arises regarding the goal of implant placement. Should the bone defect be reconstructed so the globes protrude to the same degree, or should the anatomy of the orbit be restored? My philosophy is to precisely restore the original contouring and volume of the orbit. In my experience, the most accurate means to do that is with PDS-covered titanium mesh, with precise placement and contouring as guided by MIO navigation. Globe position alone cannot be relied on—I have found that reconstruction to globe symmetry at the end of the operation leads to enophthalmos after resolution of edema. I perform exophthalmometry at the beginning and the end of the procedure to measure how far the globe is advanced as a safety check and for outcome analytics. I have found that depending on the size and location of the fracture, the globe typically advances 3 mm to 5 mm during the correction, with 2 mm to 3 mm of exophthalmos relative to the contralateral globe at the conclusion of the procedure. The majority of the edema resolves during the second and third postoperative weeks, again depending on the severity of the fracture, degree of adherence of orbital tissues to the surrounding tissue, and the duration of the procedure. The exophthalmos gradually resides during that time, but noticeable improvement in position may continue for several months.

MURR

There are abundant options regarding materials for orbital fracture repair. Certainly, for repair of rims and buttresses I prefer titanium plate and screw systems. Low-profile plates work well on the orbital rim, frontozygomatic buttress, and frontozygomaticosphenoid buttress. I believe the best options for floor reconstruction include titanium mesh, preformed titanium, porous polyethylene, titanium and porous polyethylene combinations, and autogenous material. I still prefer auricular conchal cartilage for floor reconstruction of smaller defects. Advantages of auricular cartilage include ease of harvest and location within the operative surgical field. I like that auricular cartilage is flexible yet stiff enough to support the orbital contents properly. It is the correct size and shape for all but the largest defects and, in my experience, does not need to be fixed with plates or screws. It is advantageous from a cost perspective. Porous polyethylene is a reasonable alternative but I find that the stiffness of the material can result in overcorrection with resultant globe malposition unless care is taken to be sure to place the material well posterior to the orbital rim. Otherwise, it can tent the floor contour with resultant proptosis. For larger defects where a posterior shelf is minimal or absent, I prefer the preformed titanium plates. Although computer-generated custom orbital implants are theoretically available, I have not yet taken advantage of that technology but instead have found that the preformed plates are fairly adaptable to patients. Therefore, I think they are well designed "averaged" plates. One lesson I have learned the hard way is that image guidance can be extremely important in determining that the posterior border of these essentially cantilevered plates approximates the height of the posterior floor remnant. Usually, I am trying to align the plate with the sphenoid bone. Slight differences in bend of the plate can make a big difference in the trajectory of the posterior edge. By using image guidance, I find that the plate can be accurately positioned into an optimal height when the posterior ledge is absent. I suppose intraoperative imaging can do the same thing but image guidance is certainly quicker and is as accurate, I believe. My goal is to match the contralateral globe position and approximate the volume of the orbit that would correspond to the preinjury volume. Although I do not believe that prolonged antibiotics are necessary, I usually use perioperative oral antibiotics during the surgery but frankly I cannot cite literature to support this practice. I also use perioperative corticosteroids for these cases because the corticosteroids improve postoperative edema and have a positive effect in reducing postoperative nausea. With regard to medial orbital wall fractures, I think that conchal cartilage is a suitable material. When I am confronted with orbital roof fractures, I have plated bone from the comminuted fractures back into place with low-profile thin plates and screws. One material that I do not use in the orbit is silicone. I have seen silicone sheeting become infected or erode through skin decades after placement.

WESTER

If it is a simple floor fracture, often a porous polyethylene sheet (preferably a barrier sheet with the superior nonporous surface) is used and placed securely on the posterior ledge to ensure no migration. Even for combination medial/floor fractures with an intact posterior ledge, a 0.4-mm thick nylon foil (Supramid) has been used by many with success[13] and I have used this technique or layering of these foils in smaller fractures with adequate bony support. I do not like titanium-only implants in orbital floor fracture repairs because I find these can lead to scarring and fibrosis of orbital fat and/or muscle to the implant, which can compromise motility. In cases where coated titanium plates are not available (at some off-site facilities), I place a titanium implant and then layer it with either a porous polyethylene sheet or nylon foil to minimize tissue ingrowth and scarring.

For cases of less posterior, medial, or lateral support, I often use the Medpor Titan implant. I have found the Medpor Titan 3D Orbital implant to conform nicely to the conical shape of the orbit, which is helpful in cases without a posterior ledge. The superior, nonporous barrier sheet minimizes the risk of tethering/tissue ingrowth. In complex reconstructive cases (**Fig. 4**), in particular those that are revision cases, I find customized implants of benefit. I do not typically use these implants on primary fracture cases unless they are very extensive. For a case such as that illustrated in **Fig. 4**, the patient had previous repair by another surgeon but had significant residual enophthalmos. In addition, because the rim was also fractured, a customized implant enabled cantilevering the implant from the intact lateral orbital rim. These

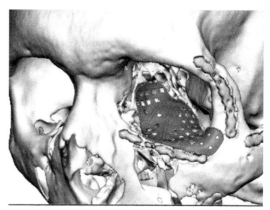

Fig. 4. 3-D CT scan demonstrating custom-manufactured titanium implant reconstructing floor and medial wall fractures.

implants (such as the KLS Martin Individual Patient Solution Orbital Implant, which uses a combination of titanium and polyether ether ketone) use volumetric analysis to compare the fractured orbit to the contralateral orbit to re-establish a more anatomic configuration to the injured side. In addition, these implants have guides for the infraorbital foramen as well as the floor to medial wall transition, which are sometimes helpful in these more difficult reconstructive cases with limited bony landmarks. The use of such navigation guides can be helpful for complex fractures, which are some of the benefits of the customized implants or 3D Titan implant, which allows for reformation of the normal slope of the inferior floor and angle between the inferior and medial wall. I have found that although the implants that require bending can be helpful when multiple normal bony landmarks are present, the premade implants are much more likely to result in optimal surgical outcomes in more complicated fractures.

The most helpful landmarks for placement of an implant depend on the extent of the fracture. When a posterior ledge is present, this allows for easy restoration of normal volume based on the superior slope to the orbital floor. When the posterior ledge is absent, I find using a preformed plate, such as the 3D Titan (I prefer the Medpor coated plates to titanium alone given the tendency of orbital tissue to adhere to the titanium) to be essential to restoring normal anatomic configuration of the orbit.

Although the ideal goal of surgical correction of an orbital fracture may be to recreate anatomy (which is often possible in simple repairs), more complex cases may not recreate normal anatomy but may achieve satisfactory results in terms of globe position, function, and aesthetic. These are the primary surgical goals for orbital floor fracture, and the use of appropriate technique and implant material is critical in success. Prophylactic sinus treatment is not necessary except in the rare case where a significant fracture may lead to a silent sinus syndrome.[14] The benefit of the customized implants in patients with a significant volumetric alteration is the ability to compare to the contralateral volume and attempt to match as closely as possible.

Question 5: How do you manage these patients postoperatively, and what surgical outcomes do you expect?

MOE

Detailed surgical consent must be obtained before surgery to repair orbital fractures, which should include a discussion of the prognosis for return of normal function as well as the risks of surgery. Included in the latter are persistent diplopia or globe malposition, eyelid malposition (ectropion and entropion), corneal damage, worsening numbness in the distribution of the infraorbital nerve, postoperative hemorrhage or retrobulbar hematoma, and diminished visual acuity or blindness (approximate risk of 0.5%).[15] These complications might require revision surgery.

Postoperatively, patients are counseled on the warning signs of retrobulbar hematoma—worsening pain, proptosis, and decreased vision—which require emergent return for evaluation. Postoperative antibiotics are not typically prescribed, given the lack of supporting medical evidence. Patients are encouraged to use iced saline gauze sponges or crushed ice packs 20 minutes per hour while awake for 48 hours and sleep with the head elevated if possible. A short course of postoperative steroids is prescribed for patients only if there is an unusual amount of edema after the repair of extensive fractures. In those cases, I also consider leaving a temporary tarsorrhaphy stitch in place for 5 days to 7 days to control chemosis. Patients are seen in follow-up 7 days to 10 days after surgery, and again 1 month, 3 months, and 12 months later if recovery is uncomplicated. Hertel measurements and visual acuity are checked at each visit, and the presence and location of diplopia is recorded. Photographs are taken at 3 months after surgery for comparison with preoperative images.

Once the acute discomfort of surgery has resolved, I instruct patients to begin physical therapy. This includes three 5-minute sessions of daily of range-of-motion exercises. Patients are instructed to hold the head stationary in neutral position and hold a finger vertically at arm's length. The patient then fixes gaze on the fingertip and moves it up, down, right, and left, stopping at the point that diplopia occurs in each direction. Effort is then made to correct the double image into a single image. I also have patients perform exercises to mobilize the orbicularis oculi muscle by forcibly closing the eye for 1 second, then opening as wide as possible for 1 second, and repeating. For patients who have had a lower lid transconjunctival approach, I also recommend gentle massage to the area, softly raising the lid vertically, obliquely toward lateral brow, and obliquely toward the medial brow to help prevent lid retraction.

Patients often ask how long to expect diplopia to persist after surgery. Unfortunately, this cannot be answered definitively due to the multiple factors that influence function. Diplopia can be caused not only by damage to bone but also by direct injury to the extraocular muscles or their innervation, ischemic damage, adhesions, and fibrosis. Repair of the fracture generally corrects the contour and volume of the orbit but not the other etiologies. Suboptimal fracture repair can lead to persistent herniation of the orbital contents as well as further entrapment of the orbital contents by an edge of the implant or adherence of orbital contents to the reconstruction material. If these factors have been ruled out, however, the diplopia resolves spontaneously in a majority of cases.[16] I have found that the incidence of postoperative diplopia is proportionate to the number of orbital walls involved with the fracture,[12] and that although most diplopia resolves within 6 weeks to 8 weeks after surgery, improvement may continue for up to a year after surgery. For patients who have diplopia that is no longer improving 3 months after surgery, I check the extraocular muscle function carefully, and if there is evidence of gaze restriction I perform forced ductions. I then also obtain a fine-cut orbital CT scan. If there is any evidence of implant malfunction (a raised edge or asymmetric contouring) on the scan, I perform an endoscopic correction. I also have the patient return to an ophthalmologist to re-evaluate the globe and muscle function. If uncorrectable neuromuscular dysfunction is diagnosed, the patient is considered for corrective muscle surgery when at least 1 year has passed after the initial surgery.

MURR

I am always on pins and needles until I can assess vision and ocular motility in the postoperative unit. I always do an early gross vision test and assess extraocular motility early. If vision is lost, opening of the wound, use of corticosteroids and Diamox, and return to the operating room for exploration are done as soon as possible. Patients are kept in house for 23 hours. Although a recent article by Kriet and colleagues[17] noted that retrobulbar hematoma as a postoperative complication is rare and postulated that outpatient surgery is feasible, I believe edema and discomfort can be better controlled in the inpatient hospital setting for the first night. Admission for 23 hours also allows the team to accomplish vision checks to be sure that if there is a change in condition, it is swiftly addressed. The first postoperative visit is typically at 1 week. Any existent skin sutures are removed at that time. Advice is given regarding scar management, specifically, use of sun protection factor 30 sunblock on the scar, massage techniques, and the use of silicone sheeting or silicone gel for scar camouflage. At this visit, a Naugle exophthalmometer is used to obtain measurements and to check globe position and projection. Often (but not always), a follow-up CT is ordered to document the surgical correction and to measure globe position. There is a low threshold to having ophthalmology follow-up, especially because the ophthalmology service evaluated the patient preoperatively. The ophthalmologists can help to determine if extraocular motility is normal. If motility is restricted, the ophthalmologists can help sort out whether persistent motility issues or diplopia is due to muscle contusion, neurologic injury, or suboptimal globe position. Any restriction of movement or diplopia warrants follow-up CT imaging.

WESTER

Outcomes of orbital fracture repair are typically good, but patient counseling preoperatively is essential (especially in cases of extensive fracture or muscle entrapment) to ensure they are aware of the potential for postoperative diplopia for several months postoperatively. Complications of fracture repair include persistent or worsening diplopia, eyelid retraction, persistent enophthalmos, blindness, mydriasis, epiphora, and implant infection or migration, risks that some investigators believe may be higher in late repair. Several steps are taken to minimize these risks. Eyelid dissection is atraumatic and through a transconjunctival approach to minimize the risk of eyelid retraction. A Frost suture is placed in the lower lid and affixed to the suprabrow area for superior lid traction after floor fracture repair. Vision, pupil, and motility are checked in the recovery room. Intraoperative hemostasis is critical and minimal pressure should be placed on the globe. Patients are sent home the same day as surgery and placed on postoperative antibiotics and a Medrol dose pack. Patients are asked to ice for the first 2 days and return in 1 week for Frost suture removal and postoperative check. They are advised to avoid excessive nose blowing.

The postoperative period is generally well tolerated. At the postoperative visits, I assess vision, motility, pupillary size and response, Hertel, infraorbital nerve sensation, and eyelid position to ensure everything is healing appropriately. With the appropriate technique, most patients heal without any visible evidence of previous surgery. Residual postoperative diplopia with a hypertropia is most commonly seen in trapdoor fractures where the inferior rectus has been entrapped at the fracture site. Patients are typically advised that this can last up to 6 months, although in my experience it often resolves within the first few weeks (depending on the time between the injury and repair). Other cases that may have persistent postoperative diplopia include reoperations where the muscle in some cases may be tethered to the implant material or cases where there is a paresis, hematoma, or fibrosis of the muscle. In addition, orbital fat atrophy can lead to persistent enophthalmos despite appropriate implant placement. In cases of persistent diplopia or enophthalmos, I advise that postoperative imaging be performed to ensure the implant is properly placed with no postoperative migration or incarceration of soft tissue.

Question 6: How have your techniques changed over the past 5 years?

MOE

My principal techniques for orbital reconstruction have not changed since 2009, when I began to use MIO-navigated reconstruction to endoscopic technique. The combination of MIO with endoscopic repair significantly improved surgical outcomes dramatically decreased the need for revision surgery. Since that time, however, I have incorporated 2 modifications that have been helpful. The first was the use of preshaped orbital implants. These are not custom-shaped to a patient's specific anatomy but are available in 2 sizes in stock, manufactured based on orbital CT scans to conform to average anatomic contours. The contours of these implants provide a good starting point for in situ adjustment to correspond with the MIO navigation plan of a patient's specific anatomy. Although these implants are commonly of insufficient size to fully span large defects, they are useful for most fractures. These are bare mesh titanium implants, and there have been multiple descriptions of adherence of orbital contents to titanium implants resulting in postoperative diplopia. As discussed preiovusly, I therefore line these implants with PDS sheeting to prevent herniation of the orbital fat through the mesh and to provide a resorbable glide layer. Functional results have been excellent using this combination in hundreds of cases.

The other recent modification to technique is the use of Hertel exophthalmometry. This has several benefits. In some cases, delineation of globe position is helpful in diagnosing asymmetry in eyelid position. It is also useful to describe to patients the difference in the position of the globes to aid in counseling patients on whether to undergo surgery, including how far the globe will be advanced and how long it might take for the globe to return to normal position and function after surgery. Intraoperative Hertel measurement is beneficial for analyzing and recording the change in orbital volume—as discussed previously, I expect 2 mm to 3 mm of exophthalmos at the end of reconstruction, depending on the site and extent of fracture. Significant deviation from this may suggest the need to reassess the accuracy of reconstruction. Postoperative measurements help describe to the patient how the healing process Is progressing and provide a highly useful tool for the surgeon to assess personal quality of outcomes.

MURR

The basics of my main technique and approach to the problem of orbital fractures were learned in residency 30 years ago. Yet, the technique has undergone nuanced evolution. The biggest change in my practice is the routine use of image guidance. This is automatic and easy for the team and it is now incorporated into the basic standard. The easy availability of sagittal CT scans is also a major change and a major advantage. The sagittal orientation can give invaluable information regarding the posterior floor shelf and also excellent views of the accuracy of the implant placement postoperatively. I was slow to adopt porous polyethylene into my practice but my oculoplastic colleagues assured me that it was safe to use, so I began using this material some years ago. As I discussed, however, I still prefer auricular conchal cartilage for smaller losses of the orbital floor. The preformed plates were released just a few years ago. I think these plates represent a significant time savings over bending the mesh in the operating room setting and for large defects I have come to depend on them. I think that in the past 5 years there has been some exuberant enthusiasm for surgically correcting medial orbital wall fractures. I have been reticent to recommend surgery for these fractures unless there is ocular dysmotility or persisting diplopia. I do not have a line out my door of patients on whom I have not operated asking me to correct their globe position problems. Finally, approximately 5 years ago I walked to the ophthalmology department and asked one of the allied health professionals to show me how to use the exophthalmometers. It was straightforward. For a couple $100 I purchased a Naugle exophthalmometer.

Having this easy-to-use tool in my outpatient clinic makes it a snap to determine globe position on a clinical basis without imaging. I think this has been one of the best advances to my practice and has helped me to be more discriminating with regard to my surgical results.

WESTER

I have found the advent of newer implant materials that allow for better anatomic re-creation advantageous in difficult cases. In addition, I have found (similar to other reports[18]) that even late surgeries can be beneficial to patients. Previously, with patients who had surgeries many years prior, I was more reluctant to perform reoperations. I have found, however, as cited by Kim and colleagues,[18] that these patients often achieve good functional and aesthetic outcomes. At the same time, fractures without clinical symptoms I am less likely to treat, because I have found conservative management is often adequate and in the rare cases of clinical symptoms developing, later intervention still leads to satisfactory results. Neobone formation and reduction of orbital volume and fracture volume can occur with time, so only those fractures that have a more significant volume impact (which can be assessed by volumetric analysis) are likely to lead to clinical symptoms. In borderline cases, waiting to assess for changes in globe position, enophthalmos and other clinical symptoms may be advantageous. Other indicators of late enophthalmos have been described to include medial wall orbital fracture size and herniated orbital fat volume in inferior orbital fractures.[19] In my practice, I have found that herniation of orbital contents (which is often but not always coexistent with fractures >50% of the floor) is the most accurate indicator of when patients are at higher risk for enophthalmos and other clinical symptoms. This was well described by Harris and colleagues[20–22] and I think is a good guide for cases of greater soft tissue displacement relative to bone fragment configuration, which may need earlier surgical intervention. In addition, the location of the fracture is important for determining time of intervention. It was recently shown that posterior medial floor fractures may demonstrate findings more similar to trapdoor fractures with improved outcomes when early intervention is performed (American Society of Ophthalmic Plastic and Reconstructive Surgery presentation, spring 2017).

REFERENCES

1. Sharma GK, Foulad A, Shamouelian D, et al. Inefficiencies in computed tomography sinus imaging

for management of sinonasal disease. Otolaryngol Head Neck Surg 2017;156(3):575–82.

2. Banerjee A, Moore CC, Tse R, et al. Rounding of the inferior rectus muscle as an indication of orbital floor fracture with periorbital disruption. J Otolaryngol 2007;36(3):175–80.

3. Chiasson G, Matic DB. Muscle shape as a predictor of traumatic enophthalmos. Craniomaxillofac Trauma Reconstr 2010;3(3):125–30.

4. Coon D, Kosztowski M, Mahoney NR, et al. Principles for management of orbital fractures in the pediatric population: a cohort study of 150 patients. Plast Reconstr Surg 2016;137(4):1234–40.

5. Scawn RL, Lim LH, Whipple KM, et al. Outcomes of orbital blow-out fracture repair performed beyond 6 weeks after injury. Ophthal Plast Reconstr Surg 2016;32(4):296–301.

6. Liao JC, Elmalem VI, Wells TS, et al. Surgical timing and postoperative ocular motility in type B orbital blowout fractures. Ophthal Plast Reconstr Surg 2015;31(1):29–33.

7. Dal Canto AJ, Linberg JV. Comparison of orbital fracture repair performed within 14 days versus 15 to 29 days after trauma. Ophthal Plast Reconstr Surg 2008;24(6):437–43.

8. Freund M, Hahnel S, Sartor K. The value of magnetic resonance imaging in the diagnosis of orbital floor fractures. Eur Radiol 2002;12:1127–33.

9. Moe KS. The precaruncular approach to the medial orbit. Arch Facial Plast Surg 2003;5:483–7.

10. Moe KS, Jothi S, Stern R, et al. Lateral retrocanthal orbitotomy; a minimally invasive canthus-sparing approach. JAMA Facial Plast Surg 2007;9(6):419–26.

11. Balakrishnan K, Moe KS. Applications and outcomes of orbital and transorbital endoscopic surgery. Otolaryngol Head Neck Surg 2011;144(5):815–20.

12. Bly R, Liu J, Cjudekova M, et al. Computer-guided orbital reconstruction improves surgical outcomes. JAMA Facial Plast Surg 2013;15(2):113–20.

13. Nunery WR, Tao JP, Johl S. Nylon foil "wraparound" repair of combined orbital floor and medial wall fractures. Ophthal Plast Reconstr Surg 2008;24(4):271–5.

14. Montezuma SR, Gopal H, Savar A, et al. Silent sinus syndrome presenting as enophthalmos long after orbital trauma. J Neuroophthalmol 2008;28(2):107–10.

15. Boyette JR, Pemberton JD, Bonilla-Velez J, et al. Management of orbital fractures: challenges and solutions. Clin Ophthalmol 2015;9:2127–37.

16. Loba P, Lozakiewicz M, Nowakowska O, et al. Management of persistent diplopia after surgical repair of orbital fractures. J AAPOS 2012;16:548–53.

17. Shew M, Carlisle MP, Lu GN, et al. Surgical treatment of orbital blowout fractures: complications and postoperative care patterns. Craniomaxillofac Trauma Reconstr 2016;9(4):299–304.

18. Kim J, Lee B, Scawn R, et al. Secondary orbital reconstruction in patients with prior orbital fracture repair. Ophthal Plast Reconstr Surg 2016;32(6):447–51.

19. Choi J, Park S, Kim J, et al. Predicting late enophthalmos: differences between medial and inferior orbital wall fractures. J Plast Reconstr Aesthet Surg 2016;69:e238–44.

20. Harris GJ, Garcia GH, Logani SC, et al. Orbital blowout fractures: correlation of preoperative computed tomography and postoperative ocular motility. Trans Am Ophthalmol Soc 1998;96:329–47.

21. Harris GJ. Orbital blow-out fractures: surgical timing and technique. Eye 2006;20:1207–12.

22. Jordan DR, St Onge P, Anderson RL, et al. Complications associated with alloplastic implants used in orbital fracture repair. Ophthalmology 1992;99:1600–8.

Evaluating New Technology

Paul J. Carniol, MD[a],*, Ryan N. Heffelfinger, MD[b], Lisa D. Grunebaum, MD[c]

KEYWORDS

- New technology • Risk/benefit technology • Lasers • Radiofrequency • ROI for technology
- Technology efficacy • Technology revenue/expenses

KEY POINTS

- One of the most important issues to consider when evaluating new technology is whether the technology will benefit patients.
- Value analysis is also imperative to the evaluation of new technology.
- The financial issues associated with acquiring new technology must also be considered.

Panel discussion

1. What is your main consideration when evaluating new technology?

2. What criteria would you use for your decision to acquire new technology?

3. How do you evaluate the efficacy of new technology before acquiring it?

4. How do you make patients aware that you have new technology?

5. How could you pay for new technology?

6. What factors affect whether new technology produces sufficient revenue to cover expenses?

Question 1: What is your main consideration when evaluating new technology?

CARNIOL

For me, the main considerations when evaluating any new technology are what it does and how effective it is. It is important that I offer my patients effective treatment options. Therefore, my first consideration is efficacy. What can the technology be used for and how effective is it? Even if there is a demand for a given technology, I only want to offer it, if there is a demonstrable result. An interesting note is, if I am not sure about a new device, I will often serve as the first patient. This practice gives me the opportunity to evaluate the treatment experience as well as the outcome.

GRUNEBAUM

I only want to endorse truly effective treatments to my patients. Regardless of potential income from a shiny and sexy new technology, if efficacy is unproven or unclear, I would not erode patients' trust in my opinion by selling treatments that may have questionable outcomes.

In my academic practice, the option for new technology investment is extremely limited. In fact, I have had one laser purchase approved in the past 7 years. For the university, the most important aspect is the business plan (return on investment [ROI]). I always downplay the business plan provided by any company, as I consistently find an individual company's income projections grossly inflated. The ROI is not the most important

---

Disclosure: The authors have nothing to disclose.
[a] Facial Plastic Surgery, Department of Otolaryngology Head and Neck Surgery, Rutgers New Jersey Medical School, 33 Overlook Road, Summit, NJ 07901, USA; [b] Division of Facial Plastic and Reconstructive Surgery, Thomas Jefferson University Hospital, 925 Chestnut Street, 7th Floor, Philadelphia, PA 19107, USA; [c] Otolaryngology/Head and Neck Surgery, University of Miami Miller School of Medicine, 1150 Northwest 14th Street, Suite 309, Miami, FL 33136, USA
* Corresponding author.
E-mail address: pcarniol@gmail.com

Facial Plast Surg Clin N Am 26 (2018) 253–257
https://doi.org/10.1016/j.fsc.2017.12.009

consideration for me as the physician. Patient trust is my most valuable asset; therefore, before I present any business plan to the university, many other aspects of a new technology are evaluated.

HEFFELFINGER

Questions that need to be addressed when evaluating new technology generally can be summarized by the following:

- What is the indication and why should I use this technology?
- How well does the new technology work? What sources of evidence are available?
- How does the evidence apply to my particular patient populations and how does it compare with the current standard?
- How can the performance of this technology be assessed, and what is an adequate time frame for assessment?

In an academic practice, the adoption rate is slow by design; everything I buy must be approved by a value analysis committee. In order to clear this committee, a purchase needs to have data that show it is clearly superior to anything else on the market for the given problem or a price that shows it is more cost-effective than the same. So, it either needs to work unbelievably well (ie, fractional carbon dioxide laser) or must be a Hermes scarf at Marshall's type of bargain (ie, used fractional carbon dioxide laser). I recommend you have your own value analysis committee, even for a process that you follow when buying technology for your office.

It is useful to decide if you are an early or a late adopter. Early adopters are on the cusp of technology and will have as many busts as they do hits. Late adopters will not consider a new technology until it is proven to work and makes complete business sense. Late adopters are okay with missing out on the next big thing and prefer to chug along on a constant, steady rate. I used to think that I wanted to be an early adopter but now put myself solidly in the latter group.

Question 2: What criteria would you use for your decision to acquire new technology?

CARNIOL

As already mentioned, the first criterion is efficacy. This criterion leads to the question of how to evaluate efficacy. I prefer to directly evaluate the technology. If the technology is approved by the Food and Drug Administration (FDA), then this evaluation can be performed by offering a free treatment with the device to some patients and observing the

outcome. Additionally, published articles in the peer-reviewed literature can also be helpful. Speaking with physicians who use the technology can also be valuable. The next criterion relates to patient demand. Is there adequate demand for this device? The next criterion is economic.[1] Is this device financially viable? First of all, can you cover the cost of the device? If you can cover the cost, can you make a profit? It does not make sense to bring a device into your practice on which you cannot at least cover all of the related expenses. Finally, does this device fit into your practice?

GRUNEBAUM

I agree with Paul but would add risk/benefit analysis. I find that patients prefer lower downtime treatments that may require multiple visits with less upside than treatments with a *wow* outcome that requires a long downtime. I also consider whether others in my community have the exact same technology. I would rather market something completely different than compete on price with my colleagues.

HEFFELFINGER

This question is a broad question with many considerations, but some pros that I like to see include the following:

- I have friends or patients who have seen improvement with the treatment by receiving treatments themselves.
- My friends or people who I really trust, preferably not doctors on the advisory board of a company or traveling trainers, have used the technology and have good things to say.
- There is good evidence in the literature that shows efficacy.

Negatives include

- The technology has been out for less than 3 years and there are not good long-term data.
- No one I know has the device.
- The science seems soft to me.
- I do not see my specific patient population spending the money on what I see as a minimal change.

Question 3: How do you evaluate the efficacy of new technology before acquiring it?

CARNIOL

In my practice, this is an important consideration. I want to perform procedures that have a demonstrable benefit to patients.

I think that, although a description of another practice's results is helpful, it is important to assess the results on my patients. Patient populations can often vary between practices. A device that works for the patients of a facial plastic surgeon in the Midwest may not be desirable for a practice in the South.

The importance of the patient demographics was demonstrated to me several years ago. It was on a rhinoplasty panel. The moderator asked how I corrected the most common nasal tip issues in my patients. Because I practice in New Jersey with a lot of Mediterranean ethnic types of noses, my immediate response was that the most common challenge was creating tip projection and definition. In my patient demographic, I treat many patients with weak, poorly defined tips. In the next seat was a surgeon from the Mayo Clinic in Minnesota who said that the most common tip problem he had to address was overprojecting tips, a completely different issue. This experience clearly demonstrated the importance and difference of patient demographics.

The possibility of variation in patient populations should be considered when speaking with another physician about a device. If you speak with another physician about the efficacy of a device, it is important to also ask about the patient population that is being treated with the device.

Another issue related to devices is how many treatments are necessary to reach the desired result. If trying a device for which more than one treatment is recommended to achieve the result, you should use it until you have performed the recommended number of treatments.

Recently, I had some sales people come into my office who suggested I should try a device on my patients. They said that at least 2 treatments should be performed. Then they told me I could only try the device once on my patients. Because this would not be an adequate trial, I declined.

After any treatment there can be swelling, ecchymoses, or pinkness, it is important to allow time to observe the result after this has resolved as part of the acute phase of recovery. I prefer to wait at least 3 to 4 weeks to assess the results of a treatment. This waiting period is important, as after some treatments there can be some swelling. Time should be allowed for this to completely resolve before assessing the response.

Your before-and-after photographs can also be helpful as part of this evaluation. It may be best to have a relatively independent evaluator review the photographs. At the least, this individual should be able to correctly identify which is before and which is after as well as rate the change.

GRUNEBAUM

I agree wholeheartedly with Paul. I like to demo a new technology in my office with trusted patients and/or staff to acquire feedback. I also discuss it with colleagues, preferably those who have some early efficacy research experience with the device (such as an initial FDA trial and so forth).

HEFFELFINGER

This evaluation is one of the most difficult things to do. Here is a scenario to avoid:

You see industry pictures that show tremendous results, so you are excited about this new technology. You speak to the representatives at multiple meetings, who introduce you to a physician who is the most experienced provider of technology X in the country.

He tells you how awesome it is. The representatives for the company arrange for you to watch a treatment at Dr I-work-for-the-laser-company's office.

The procedure seems pretty straightforward, so you decide to buy the device. The representative's ROI formula projects that you are going to make a fortune on this thing. You paid a lot but are happy to be an early adopter of the next best thing.

However, patient after patient is seeing limited results. Patients point to the picture on the brochure that you have, saying why do I not see the change like this one? You look at the fine print on the brochure, which states this patient had 7 treatment sessions. Your patient says, "7 treatment sessions, at $3000 each, that is ridiculous!" And you agree.

Question 4: How do you make patients aware that you have new technology?

CARNIOL

This question is really a marketing question. For some practices, internal marketing will be adequate. Suggest starting with internal marketing, as external marketing can be expensive. For others, external marketing will be necessary. For any directed external marketing, check that you have written consent to contact patients by e-mail or direct mail as appropriate.

GRUNEBAUM

Because of university financial constraints, my only option is my internal e-mail database. I work very hard to collect e-mails consistently from all interested patients. In addition, on occasion, after purchase of a new machine, a company may support a launch event; I advise all to take advantage of any marketing offered by industry.

HEFFELFINGER

This question points to the absolute necessity of a new practice to get the basics down first. Make sure you have optimized the patient experience from the first phone call to the last postoperative visit or your splurge on a Super Bowl commercial will fall flat as you lose patients because the people answering the phone have never heard of The Heff Lift.

I think the best marketing is free marketing, and the easiest way to market on the cheap is to cater to your captive audience. If you are in a multispecialty group or academic practice, the people buying hearing aids (ie, older patients with disposable income) are probably good candidates for what you have to offer. Forty year olds who need sinus surgery may also enjoy hearing your thoughts on different minimally invasive options for rejuvenation.

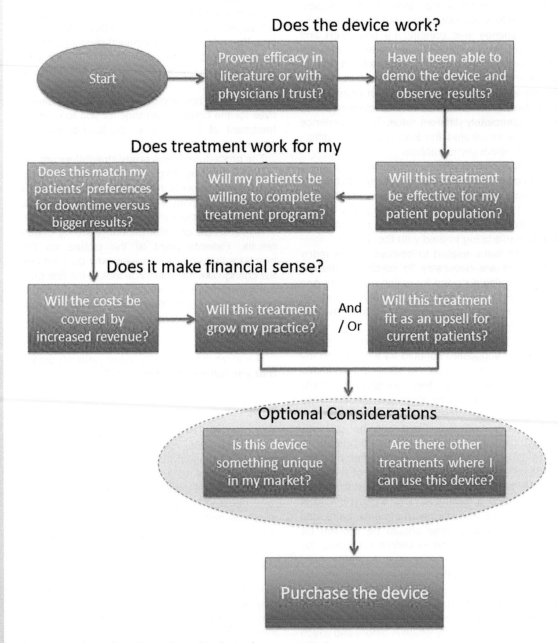

Fig. 1. Flow chart: should I purchase this device for my practice?

Investigate ways to maximize your internal marketing. For me, this is brochures throughout the office, videos played in all areas of the department/office, booths at events in the hospital cafeteria, or an afternoon lecture at a women's health event.

The next best inexpensive way to market is a little difficult but is much cheaper than hiring a marketing firm or advertising in *Big City Magazine*. Spots on television and radio are free but require a significant amount of legwork if you try to earn these on your own. Public relation (PR) firms are often less costly than marketing firms and have inside connections to TV stations, newspaper, and radio stations. My organization's PR firm has coordinated many television opportunities at a per-year rate significantly lower than the marketing firm.

Question 5: How could you pay for new technology?

CARNIOL

New technology can be purchased or leased. As underlying leasing there is financing expense, it is likely that leasing will cost more than purchasing. Also related to this question is the issue of how much you can spend on a new technology and still make a profit.

HEFFELFINGER

This question seems pretty straightforward; I am not sure there is much controversy here. What I would say is that there is a myth out there that companies are going to give you technology if you will do studies with their equipment. Not only have I found that this is not the case but there are also definite ethical dilemmas in doing this. If you get a laser for free, are you then inclined to oversell this to patients? Can you charge them

for doing it? You would be making money using a gift from industry, an obvious ethical dilemma.

Question 6: What factors affect whether new technology produces sufficient revenue to cover expenses?

CARNIOL

The factors are efficacy, competition, cost of acquisition, and cost of marketing (**Fig. 1**).

GRUNEBAUM

Can you up-sell a series? Can you up-sell associated skin care?

HEFFELFINGER

Again, this is purely a business formula. The difficult thing here is predicting how busy you will be with a given technology. For facial plastic surgeons, especially ones in academic practice, you must be careful offering treatments that are out of your specialty. It is a very slippery slide for me to start offering vaginal rejuvenation treatments in the department of otolaryngology when the obstetrics/gynecology department is a block away. So, a fat-reduction procedure that I am only using on the neck is a much worse purchase for me than it is for a general plastic surgeon who can treat multiple other areas.

REFERENCE

1. Jutkowitz E, Carniol PJ, Carniol AR. Financial analysis of technology acquisition using fractionated lasers as a model. Facial Plast Surg 2010;26(4): 289–95.

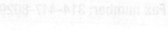
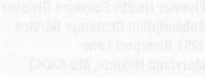

Printed and bound by CPI Group (UK) Ltd, Croydon, CR0 4YY

08/05/2025

01864711-0007